Rapid Interpretation of Heart and Lung Sounds

A GUIDE TO CARDIAC AND RESPIRATORY AUSCULTATION IN DOGS AND CATS

3251 Riverport Lane
St. Louis, Missouri 63043

RAPID INTERPRETATION OF HEART AND LUNG SOUNDS,   ISBN: 978-0-323-32707-7
THIRD EDITION
Copyright © 2015, 2006 by Saunders, an imprint of Elsevier Inc.

Notices

Knowledge and best practice in this field are constantly changing. As new research and experience broaden our understanding, changes in research methods, professional practices, or medical treatment may become necessary.

Practitioners and researchers must always rely on their own experience and knowledge in evaluating and using any information, methods, compounds, or experiments described herein. In using such information or methods they should be mindful of their own safety and the safety of others, including parties for whom they have a professional responsibility.

With respect to any drug or pharmaceutical products identified, readers are advised to check the most current information provided (i) on procedures featured or (ii) by the manufacturer of each product to be administered, to verify the recommended dose or formula, the method and duration of administration, and contraindications. It is the responsibility of practitioners, relying on their own experience and knowledge of their patients, to make diagnoses, to determine dosages and the best treatment for each individual patient, and to take all appropriate safety precautions.

To the fullest extent of the law, neither the Publisher nor the authors, contributors, or editors, assume any liability for any injury and/or damage to persons or property as a matter of products liability, negligence or otherwise, or from any use or operation of any methods, products, instructions, or ideas contained in the material herein.

Content Strategy Director: Penny Rudolph
Professional Content Development Manager: Jolynn Gower
Senior Content Development Specialist: Courtney Sprehe
Publishing Services Manager: Jeff Patterson
Senior Project Manager: Clay S. Broeker
Design Direction: Brian Salisbury
Multimedia Development: Greg Utz

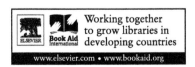

Your Complete Learning Experience!

www.heartlungsounds.com

The new, user-friendly website provides an authentic listening experience so that you are fully prepared to identify, interpret, and differentiate heart and lung sounds in dogs and cats.

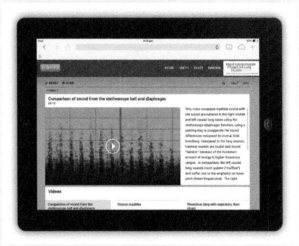

Listen and watch more than 75 heart and lung sound recordings/ videos covering murmurs, arrhythmias, and abnormal lung sounds, such as crackles, wheezes, and more.

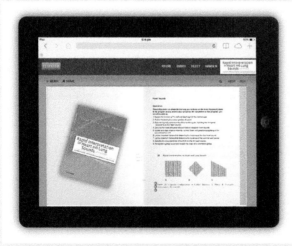

The entire text, with the sounds, videos, and tests, is integrated for ease of use.

The audio and video files are separated by topic, simplifying the ability to toggle between current and previously viewed material within the site, which facilitates review and enhances the learning process.

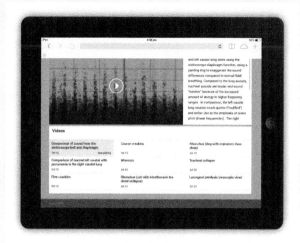

A pre-test for each chapter offers immediate feedback as you proceed through the questions.

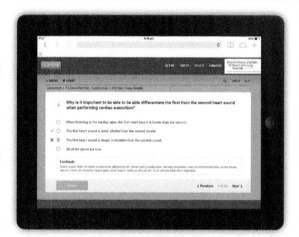

A posttest for each chapter provides a "report card" at the end of the test, allowing you to see which areas need further study and review.

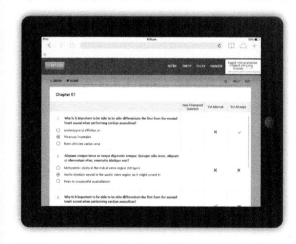

Preface

Auscultation of the heart and lungs by an expert clinician remains the most informative single diagnostic test available for the evaluation of the cardiovascular system. Auscultation presents little risk to patient or clinician, and it is quickly accomplished with inexpensive, easily maintained, highly portable equipment. Unfortunately, it takes a sustained, dedicated effort on the part of the clinician to gain substantial expertise in auscultation—and substantial expertise is needed before accurate diagnostic findings can be obtained. Auscultation potentially provides accurate information about the heart rate, rhythm, and blood flow within the heart and great vessels and may also indicate the presence and location of pulmonary pathologic conditions. Although the availability of sophisticated cardiovascular imaging methods (e.g., echocardiography, magnetic resonance imaging) has added significantly to the ability to evaluate the heart's function and anatomy, auscultation—interpreted in conjunction with a complete history and physical examination—continues to provide the key to deciding when these sophisticated diagnostic tests are appropriate. This learning package, composed of the book and a NEW companion website, is designed to help with the difficult task of acquiring expertise in auscultation.

In general, the physiology and pathophysiology of heart sounds and murmurs are similar in humans and domestic animals. A heart sound simulator was used to create most of the heart sounds in this project. The use of simulated sounds was chosen for teaching purposes because it allows the listener to focus on heart sounds without the distractions of respiratory sounds and artifacts of hair rubbing against the head of the stethoscope. Since real-life experience is also valuable, the simulated sounds are supplemented with examples taken from clinical cases. Graphic representations of electrocardiograms (ECGs) and phonocardiograms (PCGs) accompany these heart sounds for clarity and ease of understanding. Although the physiologic mechanisms responsible for heart sounds and murmurs are generally similar in humans and other animals, the heart rates, common heart diseases, conformation of the chest wall, and subsequent character of the heart sounds and murmurs when heard at the body surface are often quite different. The emphasis of this package is on heart sounds and murmurs. The material on lung sounds should be considered an introduction to this topic, with emphasis placed on material that is clearly relevant to clinical practice.

As a basis for this publication, we offer a quote from Dr. John Stone's scientific, emotional, and philosophic insights on auscultation:

> *Only with time, only after moving the stethoscope over the landscape of countless hearts, does one truly learn how to be still and listen. Such training of the ear comes only with experience. The art of auscultation is remarkably like listening to Mozart's clarinet quintet—after so long a time, one is able to follow the voice of the cello and thus appreciate its individual music within the ensemble.* (From Stone I: *In the country of hearts,* New York, 1990, Delacorte Press, p. 46.)

BRUCE W. KEENE, FRANCIS W.K. SMITH, LARRY P. TILLY, AND BERNIE HANSEN

How to Use This Learning Package

This learning package is designed to be an introduction to recognizing heart sounds, murmurs, and the auscultatory characteristics of common arrhythmias and lung sounds. We hope that it will stimulate you to continue learning by performing careful cardiac examinations and seeking out expert advice and other sources of information. Expert auscultators have built up a "mental library" of normal and abnormal sounds that they use as templates, matching the patterns and characteristics of patients' heart sounds with those in their mental libraries. It is important to examine as many hearts as possible, both normal and abnormal. Regardless of how good the quality of reproduced sounds may be, they are at best a supplement to the educational contributions of actual heart and lung sounds heard in a clinical environment under expert supervision.

Tips

- Throughout the text, two different icons—audio 🔊 and video ▶—indicate when a particular topic (e.g., First Heart Sound [S_1]) has an accompanying media file on www. heartlungsounds.com.
- To derive maximum benefit from this program, take the chapter pretest before you begin your studies. This will help you to determine how much you already know.
- Do not advance to the next chapter until you understand the material completely. Go back as often as necessary for review, and don't be afraid to move freely and repeatedly between sounds to compare subtle differences between heart sounds or murmurs that you have difficulty identifying. Emphasis must be placed on constant review and not proceeding until the material has been mastered.
- After you have completed a chapter, take the posttest (parts A and B). This will help you determine if you have mastered the material.
- In this program, some of the heart sounds and murmurs have been exaggerated to facilitate understanding of the physiologic and pathologic events. The assumption has been made that you are familiar with the physiology of blood circulation as well as with the major anatomic structures of the heart. If not, consult one of the standard cardiovascular physiology textbooks as needed.
- You should use a high-quality playback device and wear your stethoscope, holding the chestpiece of the stethoscope about 3 to 4 inches from the speaker while listening to the simulated and recorded sounds. You can also use a speaker that attaches to a laptop computer and is specifically designed for use with stethoscopes. If the sound is not transmitted through your stethoscope, you will perceive it as "booming" and less realistic.
- Many figures are used to illustrate heart sounds, murmurs, and arrhythmias. Each figure includes an electrocardiogram (ECG) situated above a phonocardiogram. The ECG is used to time heart sounds and murmurs with events (e.g., systole, diastole) in the cardiac cycle. In the phonocardiogram, single lines are used to represent heart sounds, whereas a series of lines is used to depict murmurs. The height of the lines indicates their relative intensity (loudness).

Acknowledgments

The material has been adapted from the highly regarded program for physicians titled *Rapid Interpretation of Heart Sounds and Murmurs* by Dr. Emanuel Stein and Dr. Abner J. Delman. We thank Dr. Stein and Dr. Delman for their valuable assistance in preparing this manuscript and for permitting the extensive use of figures from their text.

We appreciate the assistance of the 3M Corporation and thank Barbara Erickson, PhD, RN, CCRN, for creating the simulated heart sounds, murmurs, and arrhythmias.

We thank Caroline Miller for being our voice on the audio recordings.

We are deeply indebted to our friend, mentor, and colleague Dr. John D. Bonagura for generously contributing the clinical recordings of heart sounds, lung sounds, murmurs, and arrhythmias used on the website. Dr. Bonagura is a leading educator in veterinary cardiology, and his substantial contribution to this project has greatly enhanced its educational value.

We also acknowledge the use of some sounds from the website accompanying Dr. Steven Lehrer's *Understanding Lung Sounds,* edition 3, published by Elsevier.

A special acknowledgment goes to everyone at Elsevier—Penny Rudolph, Courtney Sprehe, Clay Broeker, and Greg Utz—for their valuable help in making this publication possible. The marketing and sales departments also must be acknowledged for generating such an interest in this book.

Contents

Resource Contents

1   Heart Sounds 🔊

- 14,000 Hz tone/10,000 Hz tone/5,000 Hz tone/1,000 Hz tone/500 Hz tone/100 Hz tone/40 Hz tone
- Transient heart sounds separated by various intervals (60 bpm [.08, .06, .04, .02])
- Normal S_1 and S_2 in the tricuspid area (60 bpm and 120 bpm)
- Splitting of S_1 in the tricuspid area (60 bpm and 120 bpm)
- S_1 in the aortic area (60 bpm and 120 bpm)
- S_1 in the mitral area (60 bpm and 120 bpm)
- Splitting of S_2 at the base of the heart (60 bpm and 120 bpm)
- Persistent splitting of S_2 (60 bpm and 120 bpm)
- Fixed splitting of S_2 (60 bpm and 120 bpm)
- Paradoxical splitting of S_2 (60 bpm and 120 bpm)
- S_3 in the mitral valve region (60 bpm and 120 bpm)
- S_4 at the left apex (60 bpm and 120 bpm)
- Atrial gallop sound in a dog
- Quadruple rhythm at the left cardiac apex (heart rate 60 bpm)
- Simulated summation gallop (120 bpm)
- Summation gallop in a cat with hypertrophic cardiomyopathy
- Aortic ejection sound in the aortic valve region as it might sound in a dog with aortic valve stenosis (60 bpm and 120 bpm)
- Midsystolic clicks in the mitral valve region (60 bpm and 120 bpm)
- Midsystolic click in a dog with mitral valve prolapse. This dog also has a sinus arrhythmia.
- Unknowns that are addressed in Posttest 1
    1. Apex.
    2. Aortic area. Identify the early systolic sound.
    3. Apex. Identify the diastolic sound. If the rate were lower, two diastolic sounds would be heard.
    4. Pulmonic area.
    5. Apex. Identify the sound following S2.
    6. Apex. Identify the midsystolic sounds.
    7. Pulmonic area. Identify the early systolic sound.
    8. Apex. Identify the sound preceding S1.
    9. Pulmonic area. This Great Dane has a normal ECG.
    10. Pulmonic area.

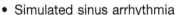

Heart Sounds

Objectives

These objectives are presented to help you to focus on the most important points in the program and to assess your progress. Upon completion of this program, you should be able to:

1. Explain the function of the bell and diaphragm of the stethoscope.
2. Outline the basic physical properties of sound.
3. Draw the hemodynamic events of the cardiac cycle, including their temporal relationship to the heart sounds.
4. Describe the basic characteristics of normal (transient) heart sounds.
5. Explain and draw what is meant by normal, fixed, and paradoxical splitting of the second heart sound.
6. List the important factors that determine the loudness of the first heart sound.
7. List the important factors that determine the loudness of the second heart sound.
8. Describe the characteristics of the third and fourth heart sounds.
9. Recognize a gallop sound and explain the origin of a summation gallop.
10. Explain the significance of an ejection sound and midsystolic click(s).

• Pretest 1

1. The first heart sound is caused by _____.
   a. closing and tensing of the left AV valve (mitral)
   b. closing and tensing of the right AV valve (tricuspid)
   c. closing and tensing of both the mitral and tricuspid valves
   d. opening of both the mitral and tricuspid valves

2. To determine the timing of cardiac events, it is important to be able to differentiate the first from the second heart sound when performing cardiac auscultation. Which of the following is true?
   a. When listening at the cardiac apex, the first heart sound is louder than the second.
   b. The first heart sound is lower pitched than the second sound.
   c. The first heart sound is longer in duration than the second sound.
   d. All of the above are true.

3. Which of the following correctly describes the timing of the heart sounds?
   a. The first heart sound occurs just after the onset of mechanical ventricular systole.
   b. The second heart sound occurs just after the onset of mechanical ventricular systole.
   c. The third heart sound occurs just after the onset of mechanical ventricular systole.
   d. None of the above is true.

4. Which of the following correctly describes the origin of a transient heart sound?
   a. The second heart sound is caused by the opening of the left and right AV valves.
   b. The third heart sound is caused by the closing of the aortic and pulmonic semilunar valves.
   c. The second heart sound is caused by the closing of the aortic and pulmonic semilunar valves.
   d. The first heart sound is caused by the opening of the aortic and pulmonic semilunar valves just after the onset of ventricular systole.

5. In dogs and cats the presence of a third or fourth heart sound is usually abnormal. These sounds are often caused by _____.
   a. rapid expansion of the aorta or pulmonary artery in early systole
   b. rapid deceleration of blood entering a stiffer than normal ventricle
   c. rapid acceleration of blood exiting a stiffer than normal ventricle
   d. rapid deceleration of blood in the aorta at the end of systole

6. A midsystolic click may indicate prolapse of the mitral valve into the left atrium, which sometimes occurs with endocardiosis of the mitral valve in dogs. Which of the following statements is true about midsystolic clicks?
   a. They are often a sign of impending heart failure.
   b. They may or may not be associated with the onset and murmur of mitral valve regurgitation.
   c. They are sometimes confused with S3 or S4, because despite their name, they can also occur during diastole.
   d. They are louder in the presence of left atrial enlargement.

7. With regard to the stethoscope chestpiece, which statement is incorrect?
   a. The diaphragm screens out some low-frequency sounds.
   b. If the bell is pressed too firmly against the chest wall, the skin may stretch and function as a diaphragm.
   c. Many heart murmurs and breath sounds sound louder and are easier to hear with the diaphragm than the bell.
   d. Gallop sounds (third and fourth heart sounds) are usually heard best with the diaphragm.

8. Choose the correct statement about gallop (third and fourth heart) sounds.
   a. They are generally lower pitched than the second heart sound.
   b. They occur during the period of ventricular diastole.
   c. At high heart rates, the period of diastole shortens, and the third and fourth heart sounds may merge to form a summation gallop sound.
   d. All of the above are correct.

9. With respect to the intensity (loudness) of transient heart sounds, choose the correct statement.
   a. The intensity of S1 depends on several factors, including the force of ventricular contraction.
   b. Decreasing systemic arterial pressures often increases the intensity of S_2.
   c. Increased pulmonary arterial pressure (pulmonary hypertension) generally decreases the intensity of S_2.
   d. All of the above are correct.

10. The quality of sound you hear with your stethoscope depends on which of the following factors?
    a. The proper application of the chestpiece to the chest wall
    b. The cleanliness of the earpieces of your stethoscope
    c. The quality and maintenance of the material of the chestpiece
    d. All of the above

Abbreviations

A_2	Aortic component of S_2	P_2	Pulmonic component of S_2
AES	Aortic ejection sound	PAT	Paroxysmal atrial tachycardia
APC	Atrial premature complex	PDA	Patent ductus arteriosus
ASD	Atrial septal defect	PES	Pulmonic ejection sound
AV	Atrioventricular	PMI	Point of maximal intensity
CCJ	Costochondral junction	PVT	Paroxysmal ventricular
cps	Cycles per second		tachycardia
DM	Diastolic murmur	S_1	First heart sound
ECG	Electrocardiogram	S_2	Second heart sound
ES	Ejection sound	S_3	Third heart sound
HOCM	Hypertrophic obstructive	S_4	Fourth heart sound
	cardiomyopathy	SM	Systolic murmur
Hz	Hertz (cycles per second,	SS	Summation sound
	a synonym of cps above)	T_1	Second main component
ICS	Intercostal space		of S_1
LBBB	Left bundle-branch block	VD	Ventrodorsal
M_1	First main component of S_1	VPC	Ventricular premature
MSC	Midsystolic click(s)		complex

Clinically Relevant Properties of Sound

Sound is produced and transmitted by vibrations. These vibrations consist of a series of waves, which are made up of compressions (areas of increased pressure) and subsequent rarefactions (areas of decreased pressure). These waves travel through solid, liquid, or gaseous media—in general, the ease and speed of transmission of sound waves are inversely proportional to the density of the media in which they are traveling. Sound waves can be fairly well described by the following physical properties.

Intensity

The intensity of sound depends on the magnitude (size or height) of the sound waves. The word we commonly use for our perception of relative sound intensity is loudness. The intensity of sound produced by a source is determined primarily by the amount of energy that goes into sound production, as well as by the efficiency of the device as a sound generator. Intensity of sound at a given location is determined by the intensity at the sound source, the distance of the listening position from the sound source (the sound intensity decreases with the square of the distance from the source—that is, if the distance from the sound doubles, the sound is only $\frac{1}{4}$ as loud), and the density and homogeneity of the media through which the sound must travel to reach the listener (sound transmission may be decreased within a medium because energy may be absorbed by the medium, and intensity may also be lost at media interfaces because of reflection).

Frequency or Pitch

The frequency of sound, also called the pitch, is determined by the number of vibrations or cycles (one compression and one rarefaction is one cycle or vibration) per second (cycles per second [cps, measured in units called hertz, or Hz]). The greater the number of cps or Hz, the higher the frequency or pitch of the sound.

Duration

The duration of a sound is the length of time the sound is produced by its source. Cardiovascular sounds include transient, short-duration vibrations (e.g., heart sounds and clicks) and may also include longer vibrations (murmurs).

Quality or Shape

The quality or shape of longer duration sounds (murmurs) is determined by the relative intensities of the individual frequency components of the murmur and their resonances (resonance in this physical sense can be thought of as the relative amplification of some frequencies within the sound) over time. This characteristic of sound can be displayed graphically as the shape or configuration of the murmur on a phonocardiogram, or sound recording. The graphic shape of the sound (a depiction of the intensity and frequency of the sound over time) is associated with a quality of sound the ear can be trained to recognize, much in the way that an oboe playing the same note at the same intensity as a clarinet is still recognizable as an oboe.

Perception of Sound

In addition to the physical properties of sound, which are dictated by the circumstances of its production and transmission, our perception of cardiovascular sounds is also influenced by the sensory and integrative mechanisms involved in hearing. The perceived intensity (loudness or softness) of sound is influenced by both the actual physical intensity of the sound (i.e., the magnitude of the sound waves) and its frequency. This is because human hearing is not equally responsive to sound in all frequency ranges. A sound in the ear's optimal sensitivity range (1000 to 5000 cps) will be perceived as being louder than an equally intense but lower frequency sound (e.g., 200 Hz) because of the ear's relatively poor sensitivity to sounds in the lower frequency range. Even among individuals with "normal" hearing, there is some potentially important variability in hearing sensitivity, especially in the low end of the frequency range.

> ✳ **KEY POINT** Loudness, the perceived intensity of a sound, is influenced by the frequency of the sound.

In addition to inherent individual variability in hearing sensitivity, wide and clinically important, measurable differences in hearing occur as the result of training. These differences involve the ability to correctly perceive the shape or quality of sounds, as well as the ability to distinguish two transient sounds separated by a brief period of time as separate sounds. In this regard, individuals who have undergone serious musical training or who speak a language having multiple meanings and pronunciations of the same phoneme (e.g., Cantonese) in addition to English have a significant advantage.

Cardiovascular Sounds

Most cardiovascular sounds are produced in the heart and great vessels and transmitted through liquid, solid, and gaseous media to the chest wall. We generally use a stethoscope to transmit the cardiovascular sounds from the chest wall to our ears. Cardiovascular sounds can be divided into brief, circumscribed sounds (so-called transient sounds, which include heart sounds and clicks), and longer combinations of vibrations (heart murmurs).

Almost all clinically significant cardiovascular sounds occur in the frequency range of 20 to 500 cps (occasionally up to 1000 cps). The transient heart sounds heard most commonly in dogs and cats can be divided into (1) normal sounds (the first and second heart sounds, S_1 and S_2); (2) normal and abnormal variations of S_1 and S_2; (3) diastolic heart sounds that usually reflect the presence of cardiac disease, such as S_3 and S_4 (gallop sounds); and (4) systolic ejection sounds or clicks (ESs) and midsystolic or late-systolic clicks (MSCs) that may or may not indicate the presence of significant heart disease. Heart murmurs are longer, more complex sounds.

Auscultation of the heart is limited by two factors. First is the threshold sensitivity of the human ear. The normal adult can detect sound frequencies from around 20 to 14,000 Hz, but the ear is most efficient in the frequency range from 1000 to 5000 Hz. Below 1000 Hz, auditory sensitivity progressively decreases, impairing the ability to hear and accurately judge the intensity of sounds in this frequency range (some of these sounds can actually be better felt with the hand as vibrations). Thus an intense cardiovascular sound in this low-frequency range may be perceived as a soft sound that is difficult to hear. The relationship between the range of human hearing and cardiovascular sound is shown in Figures 1-1 and 1-2. The temporal relationship between heart sounds is also important. The human ear can normally identify two sounds separated by between 0.02 and 0.03 second as two distinct sounds. Two sounds separated by less than 0.02 second are thus most often heard as a single sound. Because of this lack of "acoustical acuity," appreciation of a split heart sound or differentiation of two closely coupled sounds as distinct sounds requires that the sounds be separated by at least 0.02 second. With practice, the human ear can be trained

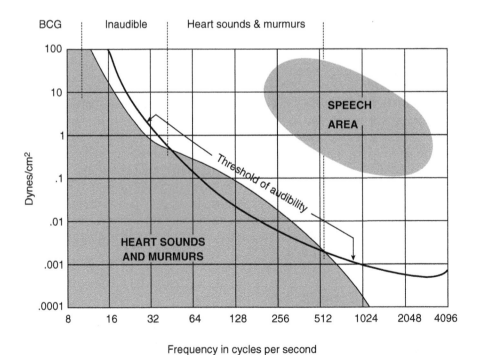

Figure 1-1 Common frequency ranges of heart sounds and murmurs. *(From Butterworth JS et al: Cardiac auscultation, New York, 1960, Grune & Stratton.)*

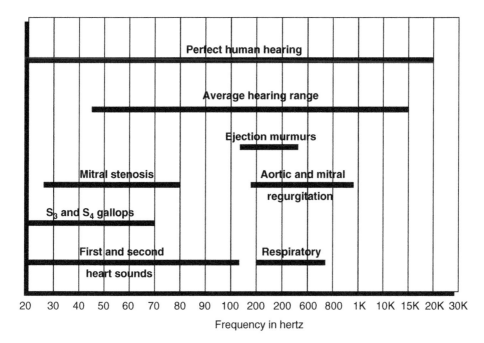

Figure 1-2 Relative frequency ranges. Note that this figure does not depict sound intensity or loudness. *(From Selig MB: Stethoscopic and phonoaudio devices: historical and future perspectives. Am Heart J 126:262, 1993.)*

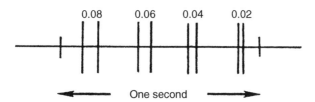

Figure 1-3 **Various intervals (in hundredths of a second).**

to more accurately recognize sounds that are separated by brief time intervals as distinct sounds. Some heart sounds that are commonly appreciated as containing two distinct components (split sounds) in humans (e.g., physiologic splitting of S_2 with inspiration) are more difficult to appreciate as distinct sounds in dogs and cats because of their relatively high heart rates and inability to cooperate (e.g., by taking a deep breath). Several examples of intervals between closely coupled sounds are depicted in Figure 1-3 and demonstrated on the accompanying website. The stethoscope itself may also impose limitations on auditory acuity.

Stethoscope

The main components of the stethoscope are the chestpiece (bell and diaphragm, which come in contact with the chest wall), tubing (connects the chestpiece to the binaural

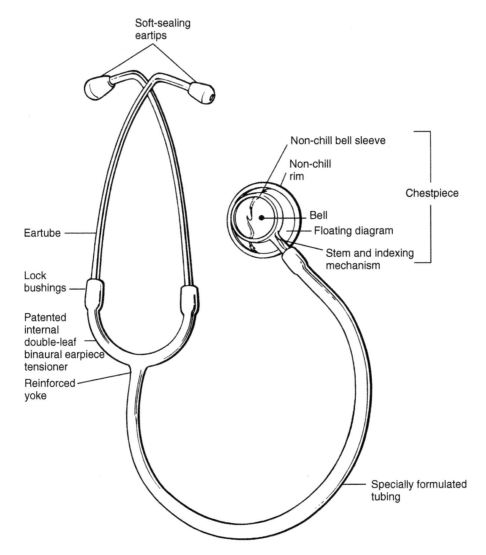

Figure 1-4 Anatomy of a stethoscope with a combination chestpiece. Chestpieces are available in several sizes. A pediatric or infant chestpiece is often recommended for cats and small dogs.

headpiece), binaural headpiece (distributes the sound to each ear), and earpiece tips (Figure 1-4). The bell of an efficient stethoscope when held lightly against the chest wall transmits all sounds produced within the chest, both low (20 to 100 Hz) and higher frequencies (100 to 1000 Hz), with little attenuation. Intense (loud) low-frequency components of a mixed-frequency sound may "mask out" the high-frequency components of the murmur, so that the high-frequency components may be perceived as faint or absent when heard with the bell. The diaphragm of the stethoscope applied firmly to the chest wall is designed to attenuate (filter out) low frequencies (20 to 100 Hz) and selectively transmit higher frequencies so they can be better heard. The best diaphragm materials are moderately stiff and resist cracking when dropped onto hard surfaces. Most stethoscopes feature a bell and

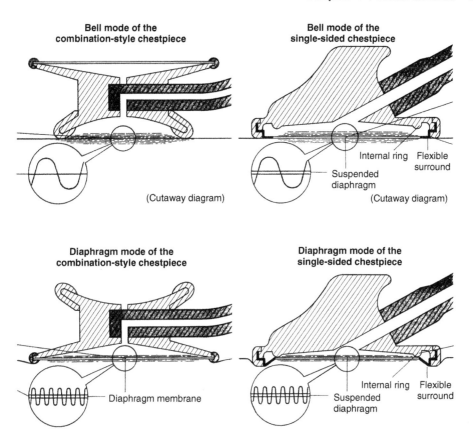

Figure 1-5 The stethoscope on the left is the traditional design with separate bell and diaphragm (combination-style chestpiece). The stethoscope on the right, the 3M Littmann Master Classic 2™ Stethoscope, is a newer design that incorporates the bell and diaphragm into a single head (single-sided chestpiece). Light pressure produces the effect of the bell, and increased pressure produces a diaphragm response. *(Courtesy of 3M Health Care, St. Paul, Minn.)*

a diaphragm separated by a bearing that allows each individual component to be locked into place in perfect alignment with the tubes. The quality and durability of the bearing and mechanism that align the bell or diaphragm to the tubing are the single biggest determinants of the life expectancy of these stethoscopes.

A stethoscope design by 3M combines the bell and diaphragm into one, single-sided chestpiece. The Littmann "Master" series stethoscopes use a single-sided chestpiece design that combines both the bell and the diaphragm modes onto the same side of the chestpiece (Figure 1-5). Varying fingertip pressure allows the user to switch from a chestpiece that emphasizes low-frequency (light pressure) or high-frequency (firm pressure) sounds. This chestpiece design is more convenient and efficient for auscultation than a traditional two-sided stethoscope, because switching from bell to diaphragm does not interrupt auscultation. The potential acoustical drawback of the design is that the diaphragm material cannot be completely removed from the sound path when the "bell function" of the instrument is being used.

The tube(s) of the stethoscope connect the chestpiece with the binaural earpieces. Tubing should be flexible, smooth, and thick walled to reduce ambient noise and optimize sound transmission. Shorter tubing causes less attenuation of high-frequency sounds. For ideal high-frequency sound transmission, two separate tubes should connect the chestpiece with the binaural earpieces (the two tubes may be wrapped together or housed in a larger tube from the chestpiece up to the level of the binaural headpiece to keep the tubes from bumping together). A practical tubing length is approximately 12 to 20 inches. The binaural headpiece should hold the earpieces at a comfortable distance apart, and the tension should be adjustable to accommodate a variety of head sizes. The earpieces should curve gently forward, in the direction of the ear canal. The magnitude of this forward curve should also be somewhat adjustable by rotation of each earpiece within its respective tube at the base of the binaural headpiece. Cleanable, replaceable earpiece tips should be comfortable and occlude the ear canal without entering the canal. Many types and sizes of earpiece tips are available. The most appropriate earpiece tips for any listener are best determined by trial and error. Proper forward angulation and tensioning of the earpieces combined with comfortable earpiece tips are essential for optimal auscultation.

Electronic stethoscopes have improved dramatically, but even with "noise cancellation" technology, electronic amplification of ambient background noise along with the heart sounds remains problematic. This problem can be partially addressed by coupling the electronic stethoscope's chestpiece to the chest wall with carefully applied ultrasound gel (the stethoscope must be cleaned thoroughly after each use when this is done, and some care is needed to make sure that there are no breaks in the covering of the electronics that might allow gel or moisture to enter the device). In addition to electronic amplification of heart sounds and murmurs, most of the electronic stethoscopes currently allow the user to record and play back sounds at either normal or half speed, a useful feature for judging the timing and shape or quality of murmurs in tachycardic patients and for judging the timing of transient heart sounds such as clicks or gallops. Some models also provide the ability to record graphic representations of sounds in a digital file format (i.e., a phonocardiogram) that can be stored on a computer, potentially becoming part of the patient's medical record. An extra-cost option for the Welch Allyn Meditron electronic stethoscope provides hardware and software that allow simultaneous recording of an electrocardiogram (ECG), with subsequent transfer of the files to a computer for storage of the phonocardiogram, complete with ECG timing and sound. The 3M Littmann models that feature ambient noise reduction circuitry appear to reduce background noise by approximately 75% without significantly filtering body sounds. These stethoscopes have the additional advantage of allowing wireless digital file transfer to a computer.

Keys to Successful Auscultation

A clean (unobstructed), properly fitted and functioning stethoscope is of great importance in the thorough examination of the heart and lungs. The earpieces must be large enough to fit snugly without entering the ear canals. The chestpiece should consist of a bell and a diaphragm in either a combination style or a single-sided version. Appropriate use of the bell or diaphragm is critical to accurate auscultation. Although the bell transmits all the sounds coming from the chest with the least attenuation, it is best used to hear low-frequency sounds and murmurs because these low-frequency sounds may mask the presence of high-frequency murmurs. The bell should be applied with light pressure on the chest wall—just enough pressure to seal out room noise. Too much pressure on the bell tightens the skin beneath it and creates a sort of diaphragm that filters out the lower frequencies.

⁑ **KEY POINT** Always use the bell and diaphragm for optimal auscultation of low- and high-frequency sounds, respectively.

The diaphragm is designed to screen out low-frequency sounds and should be applied firmly to the chest wall (firmly enough to leave a ring on your hand for a few seconds after you remove it) to closely couple the head of the stethoscope to the chest wall. Extra care is required when listening to puppies and kittens with the diaphragm, because excessive chest pressure may create murmurs in small or thin-chested animals. The most commonly observed and clinically important stethoscope problems include the presence of air leaks (e.g., cracked diaphragm, tubing, or earpiece tips that allow infiltration of outside air into the system), partially obstructed earpieces, improper alignment of the chestpiece with the tubes (malfunction of the chestpiece bearing), and improper alignment of the earpieces with the ear canals (e.g., putting the stethoscope on "backwards"). Even a small crack in the diaphragm can reduce sound transmission dramatically—and replacing a cracked diaphragm with a piece of x-ray film does not solve the problem.

⁑ **KEY POINT** Always use light pressure with the bell, because firm pressure will create the effect of a diaphragm.

The physical examination is best accomplished with a quiet patient in a quiet room—two commodities that may be in short supply under clinical circumstances. Loud room ventilation, intrusive hallway noise, barking, purring, panting, and persistent client conversation are all potential impediments to successful auscultation. The patient should be standing, preferably on a table unless the animal is too big. It is helpful to have an assistant hold the patient's head gently but firmly away from the assistant's body (to avoid having to deal with a sniffing patient) and close the patient's mouth if the patient is panting constantly.

Each cardiovascular examination should begin with palpation of the precordium (the area of the chest wall that overlies the heart and great vessels), with the examiner's hands flat on each side of the patient's chest wall. Palpation of the precordial cardiac impulse defines the approximate location of the heart in the chest and may provide valuable clues to cardiac enlargement (dilation or hypertrophy) and function. Murmurs of sufficient intensity produce palpable vibrations on the precordium called thrills, which reliably localize the point of maximal intensity of the murmur. The cardiac rhythm can also be assessed in this way, as can the compressibility of the thorax (in cats).

After palpation of the precordium, the arterial pulses are evaluated bilaterally, usually at the femoral artery, to assess the heart rate, rhythm, and arterial pulse quality. The arterial pulse pressure is the difference between the systolic and diastolic arterial pressure. The arterial pulse quality varies with body condition, species, age, heart rate, hydration, intravascular volume status, ventricular function, and level of excitement or activity. Hyperkinetic pulses (stronger than normal) can be caused by any condition that augments the stroke volume or rate of ejection of blood from the left ventricle (e.g., volume loading of the left ventricle) or decreases the diastolic pressure in the arterial system or both. Common conditions associated with hyperkinetic pulses include fever, hyperthyroidism, aortic regurgitation, and patent ductus arteriosus. Hypokinetic pulses (weaker than normal) are often associated with reduced intravascular volume, shock, heart failure, or aortic stenosis.

Variable-intensity pulses are often a sign of arrhythmia (e.g., atrial fibrillation). A special case of variable-intensity pulses, called pulsus paradoxus, is associated with pericardial disease and elevated intrapericardial pressures. Pulsus paradoxus is defined by a peripheral arterial pulse pressure that decreases palpably (by more than 10% to 15%) with inspiration.

A systematic approach to cardiac auscultation optimizes recognition and categorization of any abnormalities present. After palpation of the precordium and arterial pulses, the chestpiece of the stethoscope is placed over the cardiac apex (at the point of maximum impulse). The normal cadence of S_1 and S_2 (lub-dup, where "lub" is S_1 and "dup" is S_2) is identified first—at the cardiac apex, S_1 should normally be louder, longer, and lower pitched than S_2. Care must be taken to identify the origin of potentially confusing sounds that commonly arise as a result of breathing, shivering, twitching, or movements of the stethoscope diaphragm against the hair coat. Venous hum, sometimes audible at the thoracic inlet, can also be confused with a heart murmur, and routine auscultation in this location is fraught with potential error. Noises originating in finger joints may also cause problems, and examiners need practice in keeping the hand still and silent on the chestpiece.

During auscultation the chestpiece is repositioned several times as the auscultator moves it slowly between the apex and the heart base, listening over the entire precordium on the left hemithorax, including the area deep in the armpit. This procedure, called "inching" the stethoscope, is repeated on the right hemithorax, first with the diaphragm of the stethoscope, and then the process is repeated with the chestpiece switched to the bell. As auscultation moves from the apex toward the heart base, in normal animals S_2 becomes progressively louder (and S_1 softer) until the diaphragm reaches the heart base, where S_2 is louder and higher pitched than S_1. The change in relative intensities of S_1 and S_2 can be represented as follows: moving from the apex (LUB-dup), to midway between the apex and base (lub-dup), to the heart base (lub-DUP). Conditions that uniformly alter the loudness of heart sounds are listed in Box 1-1.

✳ **KEY POINT** Inching the stethoscope from the cardiac apex to the heart base helps differentiate S_1 (loudest at the apex) from S_2 (loudest at the base).

After identifying the cadence of S_1 and S_2 at each location on the chest wall, the auscultator should concentrate on describing any other sounds or murmurs that might be present.

▪ **Box 1-1 Conditions That Alter Loudness of All Heart Sounds**

Increase Loudness
Thin-chested animals
Vigorous ventricular contraction (hyperthyroidism, excitement)

Decrease Loudness
Obesity
Pleural effusion
Pericardial effusion
Diaphragmatic or pericardial diaphragmatic hernia
Pneumothorax
Decreased ventricular contraction (hypothyroidism, dilated cardiomyopathy)

These descriptions must include their point of maximal intensity (where the sound is best heard), intensity (loudness on a scale of 1 to 6 for murmurs), timing (when the sound is heard), duration (how long the sound lasts), and quality (the shape of the sound). Murmurs and their description are discussed in detail in Chapter 2. The effects of respiration on the heart rhythm, heart sounds, and any murmurs present should be noted.

Palpating a peripheral artery while auscultating the heart can aid in identifying the first heart sound (the arterial pulse rises immediately after S_1) in patients whose normal cadence of S_1 and S_2 (lub-dup) is difficult to identify. Simultaneous auscultation and arterial pulse palpation can also potentially identify pulse deficits (S_1s that are not accompanied by the upstroke of an arterial pulse and also not followed by normal S_2s). Pulse deficits generally indicate the presence of a cardiac arrhythmia and often accompany premature beats (either ventricular or supraventricular) at high heart rates. Simultaneous auscultation and pulse palpation can be confusing, however, not infrequently resulting in unwarranted concern over the presence of arrhythmias in otherwise healthy, asymptomatic animals with heart rates less than 120 beats per minute. It is important to remember that pulse deficits are unlikely to occur, even in the face of ectopic beats, at low or normal heart rates. It's also worth remembering that no matter what we may think of our skills, our brains are not great at multitasking!

Principal Areas of Cardiac Auscultation

Frequent reference will be made to the four primary valve areas illustrated in Figure 1-6 and listed in Table 1-1. Additional areas are also essential in cardiac auscultation.

✳ **KEY POINT** Auscultate over all four valve regions, especially in puppies and kittens.

Hemodynamics of the Cardiac Cycle

Understanding the hemodynamics of the cardiac cycle (illustrated in Figure 1-7) is critical to making sense of cardiac auscultation. The cardiac cycle is continuous, of course, but it is useful to think about the events of sequential contraction and relaxation as traditionally divided into two time periods.

▪ **Table 1-1** Principal Areas of Cardiac Auscultation

	Dog	**Cat**
Mitral area	L 5 ICS at CCJ	L 5-6 ICS, $\frac{1}{4}$ VD distance from sternum
Aortic area	L 4 ICS above CCJ	L 2-3 ICS just dorsal to pulmonic area
Pulmonic area	L 2-4 ICS at left sternal border	L 2-3 ICS, $\frac{1}{3}$-$\frac{1}{2}$ VD distance from sternum
Tricuspid area	R 3-5 ICS near CCJ	R 4-5 ICS, $\frac{1}{4}$ VD distance from sternum

CCJ, Costochondral junction; *ICS*, intercostal space; *VD*, ventrodorsal.

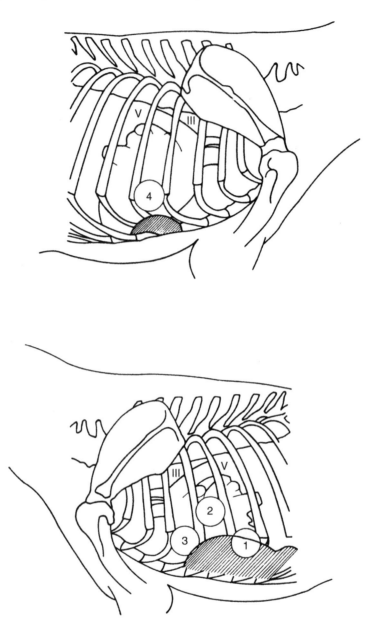

Figure 1-6 Principal areas of cardiac auscultation in the dog. The valve relationships are the same in the cat. *1*, Mitral valve area; *2*, aortic valve area; *3*, pulmonic valve area; *4*, tricuspid valve area. Mitral, aortic, and pulmonic valves are auscultated on the left hemithorax. The tricuspid valve is auscultated on the right hemithorax. *Shaded area*, Area of cardiac dullness. *(From Detweiler D, Patterson DF: A phonograph record of the heart sound and murmurs of the dog. Ann NY Acad Sci 127:323, 1965.)*

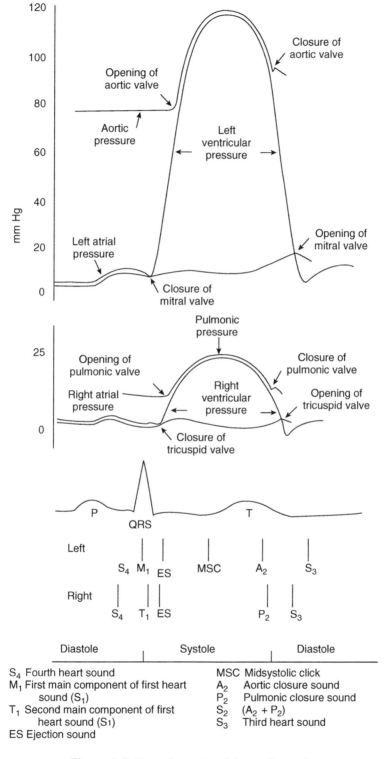

Figure 1-7 Hemodynamics of the cardiac cycle.

Ventricular Systole

The ventricles begin to contract after they have been electrically activated (electrical activation of both ventricles is recorded as the QRS complex of the ECG). As soon as contraction of the ventricular muscles raises the pressure inside the ventricular chambers above that in the atria (generally less than 10 mm Hg), the mitral and tricuspid atrioventricular valves close and tense (causing both the mitral [M_1] and tricuspid [T_1] components of the first heart sound, S_1). S_1 provides an audible signal of the beginning of mechanical ventricular systole. A brief period of systole, isovolumetric contraction, ensues in which the pressure in the ventricles increases but the ventricular volume remains constant. The systolic period of isovolumetric contraction ends when the pressure inside the ventricles reaches the pressure in the aorta and pulmonary artery, such that the aortic and pulmonic semilunar valves open and the ejection phase of systole begins. The ejection phase of the cardiac cycle is subdivided into an early, brief phase of rapid ejection (a period of rapid rise in the aortic and ventricular pressures accompanied by the rapid ejection of blood from the ventricles) and a somewhat longer phase of reduced ejection. The entire period of ejection is normally silent (all normal heart valves open silently, and the flow of blood from the ventricles into the aorta and pulmonary arteries is smooth and noiseless, or laminar). Throughout the period of ventricular systole, blood continues to return to the atria and atrial pressures rise progressively. By the end of ventricular muscle contraction (systole), the normal ventricle in the dog or cat has ejected well over half of the blood that was present at the beginning of systole. The difference between the volume in the ventricle at the beginning of systole (actually the end of the preceding period of diastole) and the volume present at the end of systole is known as the stroke volume, and the fraction of blood ejected from the ventricle is called the ejection fraction.

Ventricular Diastole

At the end of systole the ventricular pressures fall, and as soon as the pressures fall below the pressures in the aorta and pulmonary artery, the aortic and pulmonic valves close (causing the second heart sound, S_2). S_2 is subdivided into an aortic component (A_2) and a pulmonic component (P_2) and provides an audible marker for the end of systole and the beginning of diastole. Analogous to the beginning of systole, in diastole a brief period of isovolumetric relaxation occurs. During this brief time the ventricular muscles are actively relaxing and the pressure in the ventricles falls whereas their volume does not change (both atrioventricular [AV] and semilunar valves are closed). When the ventricular pressures fall below the atrial pressures, the period of rapid ventricular filling begins and blood rushes into the ventricles through the open mitral and tricuspid valves. As with ejection, blood flowing into the ventricles is normally a silent event. Ventricular volume rises rapidly during this phase, and atrial pressures decrease. In horses and cows (large animals with large ventricles) or dogs and cats with excessively stiff ventricles, rapid deceleration of blood associated with the end of the rapid filling phase can result in a transient, low-frequency third heart sound (S_3).

The rapid filling phase is followed by a phase of slow ventricular filling called diastasis. During diastasis, additional passive ventricular filling occurs and there is a gradual (and normally small) increase in both atrial and ventricular pressures. Atrial contraction begins just after electrical activation of the atria (the P wave of the electrocardiogram); atrial systole (which occurs during ventricular diastole) results in a boost (up to 30% at high heart rates) to ventricular volume; and atrial and ventricular pressures both rise a bit. In many normal horses and cows, as well as in dogs or cats with abnormally stiff ventricles, a transient, low-frequency fourth heart sound (S_4) may be associated with the deceleration of blood entering the ventricles after atrial systole, immediately before the onset of ventricular systole.

First Heart Sound (S_1)

We begin our study of the first heart sound by listening over the mitral area (left cardiac apex) to the characteristic "LUB-dup" cadence of the normal heart sounds at this location. S_1, which signals the onset of ventricular systole (see Figure 1-7), can be heard well with both the bell and the diaphragm of the stethoscope. M_1 and T_1, the two main components of S_1, however, have predominantly higher frequency vibrations, which are best appreciated with the diaphragm. The main component of S_1, the mitral component (M_1), is typically heard loudest at the left cardiac apex. M_1 represents energy vibrations released from the abrupt closing and tensing of the mitral valve apparatus early in ventricular systole. Audible variations in the intensity (loudness) of S_1 are usually caused by alterations in M_1.

> ✳ **KEY POINT** S_1 is heard best with the diaphragm over the area of the left cardiac apex.

The second main component of S_1, the tricuspid component (T_1), is usually softer than M_1 and is heard best at the tricuspid area (right cardiac apex). T_1 is caused by the tricuspid valve closing and tensing early during right ventricular systole. Physiologic splitting of S_1 (audible separation of M_1 and T_1 without an identifiable pathologic cause) is rarely appreciated in dogs and cats. It is heard occasionally as a normal variant in large and giant breeds of dogs. Pathologic splitting of S_1 is most often a result of ventricular conduction disturbances that delay the electrical activation of one ventricle (bundle-branch blocks) or of ventricular ectopic beats (ventricular premature complexes [VPCs] or ventricular escape complexes), in which the ventricle where the ectopic focus resides may be activated significantly before the other ventricle. When present, audible splitting of S_1 is generally best appreciated in the tricuspid area (Figure 1-8). Even when the split is audible in the tricuspid area, S_1 may be heard as a single sound on the left hemithorax (Figures 1-9 and 1-10). A split S_1 must be differentiated from an S_4-S_1, S_1–ejection sound, and S_1–systolic click.

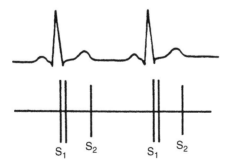

Figure 1-8 Mitral and tricuspid components of S_1 (split sounds) and S_2 in the tricuspid area. Note that S_1 is louder than S_2 in the tricuspid area. Rarely, S_1 is heard as a split sound in the tricuspid valve area in giant-breed dogs.

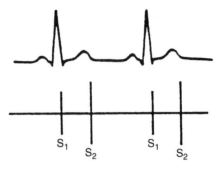

 Figure 1-9 S_1 **and** S_2 **in the aortic area.** Note that S_2 is louder than S_1 in the aortic area.

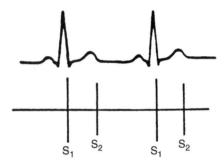

Figure 1-10 S_1 **and** S_2 **at the left apex.** Note that S_1 is louder than S_2 at the left apex.

The relative and absolute intensity (loudness) of S_1 at the cardiac apex may provide the astute auscultator with some insight into the structure and function of the heart. The examiner first compares the intensity of S_1 with that of S_2 because many conditions alter the loudness of all heart sounds (see Box 1-1). An absolute assessment of the appropriateness of the intensity of S_1 for the patient and circumstances is needed, however, because some conditions affect the intensity of S_2 independent of S_1 (i.e., it is generally unsafe to assume that a large differential in the relative intensity of S_1 and S_2 has been caused by a change in the intensity of S_1). In normal animals the apparent intensity of S_1 ranges from approximately half to twice that of S_2, depending on the listening location. Most often, S_1 is appreciated as louder, longer, and lower pitched than S_2 when heard in the mitral area (left cardiac apex). The normal "LUB-dup" pattern or cadence heard here usually consists of a single S_1 sound and a single S_2 sound (usually reflecting predominantly M_1 and A_2).

✳ **KEY POINT** Two common diseases in cats, systemic hypertension and hyperthyroidism, can cause an accentuated S_1.

Analogous to slamming a door, the intensity of S_1 depends on the force with which the mitral valve is closed as well as the relative position of the open valve leaflets when that force is applied (and to a lesser degree, the health of the valve tissue itself). With respect to the door analogy, it is easy to see that a door must be open more than a crack when slammed to make the loudest possible noise, that the noise will be louder when the person doing the slamming puts some serious muscular effort into the event, and that a door made from stout stuff will make a bigger noise when struck forcefully by the jamb. The intensity

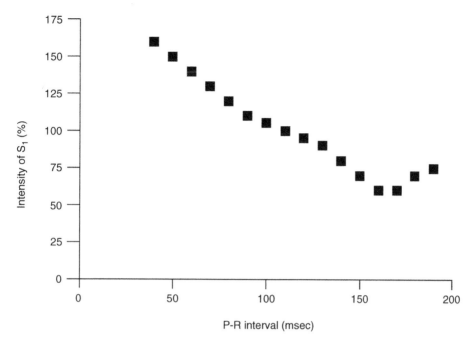

Figure 1-11 Graph demonstrating relationships between loudness of S_1 with varying P-R intervals.

of S_1 reflects the force behind valve closure (ventricular contraction), which is determined by the contractile state of the ventricle, as well as the volume status of the patient (remember the Frank-Starling law). Conditions that reduce contractility or ventricular volume (e.g., beta-blocking drugs or hypovolemic shock, respectively) often reduce the absolute, and potentially the relative, intensity of S_1. In addition to the force of contraction, the position of the mitral valve at the beginning of ventricular contraction is an important determinant of the intensity of S_1. For the same effort (force) a louder noise will be made when the valve leaflets have farther to travel before they are slammed shut. The valve position at the end of ventricular diastole is determined primarily by the P-R interval of the ECG. For example, if the P-R interval is short (as in ventricular preexcitation), the atria will contract immediately before ventricular contraction, forcing the valves wide open before ventricular contraction and creating a loud S_1; conversely, if the P-R interval is long (e.g., first-degree AV block), the valves are opened normally after atrial contraction but drift closer together again when ventricular contraction is not immediately forthcoming, reducing the intensity of S_1. Thus the loudest S_1 for any given force of contraction occurs when the P-R interval is short; most "in-between" P-R intervals result in an S_1 of midrange intensity; and a relatively soft S_1 may be produced by long P-R intervals. The relationship between the intensity of S_1 and the P-R interval for any given volume and contractile state is shown in Figure 1-11. Potential causes of either abnormally accentuated or diminished first heart sounds are listed in Boxes 1-2 and 1-3.

In addition to being abnormally loud or soft, S_1 can vary dramatically in intensity from beat to beat with varying P-R intervals or with marked variations in the R-R interval as seen with atrial fibrillation, pronounced sinus arrhythmia, Mobitz type I second-degree AV block, and atrial or ventricular premature beats.

■ **Box 1-2** Abnormally Accentuated S_1

Short P-R interval
Vigorous left ventricular contraction
    Pregnancy
    Hyperthyroidism
    Exercise
    Fever
    Anemia
    Systemic hypertension
    Inotropic agents (e.g., epinephrine)
    Excitement or fear
    Arteriovenous fistula

■ **Box 1-3** Abnormally Diminished S_1

Prolonged P-R interval (first-degree AV block)
Diminished left ventricular function
    Hypothyroidism
    Severe congestive heart failure—dilated cardiomyopathy
    Shock (hypovolemic)
    Left bundle-branch block
    Negative inotropic agents (e.g., beta blockers)
Abnormal isovolumetric contraction
    Aortic regurgitation
    Mitral regurgitation
Heavy calcification or destruction of the mitral valve

Second Heart Sound (S_2)

We now shift our auscultation from the cardiac apex to the base. S_2 is normally louder than S_1 when heard at the base of the heart (the cadence here is lub-DUP). S_2 is also shorter in duration, and higher in pitch (frequency) than S_1. S_2 marks the termination of ventricular systole, as diagrammed in Figure 1-7. S_2 is composed of two components, aortic (A_2) and pulmonic (P_2), and these individual components may be audible in normal animals because of asynchronous closure of first the aortic and then the pulmonic valve. The audibility of this split is greatly (and physiologically) enhanced during inspiration, when intrathoracic pressure and pulmonary vascular resistance fall and venous return increases to the right ventricle, while pooling of blood in the lungs decreases venous return to the left ventricle. As a result, right ventricular ejection time is prolonged, with a delay in P_2, and left ventricular ejection time is shortened, with earlier occurrence of A_2. Physiologic splitting of S_2 is difficult to detect in dogs and cats with high respiratory or heart rates. A_2 is usually audible over all the standard areas of cardiac auscultation and is best heard at the aortic and pulmonic areas. P_2 is normally softer than A_2 and is usually heard best at the pulmonic area (left heart base). Therefore separation of S_2 into its two components, when possible, is best perceived at the left heart base just after inspiration. At the mitral area, S_2 is usually heard as a single sound (Figure 1-12).

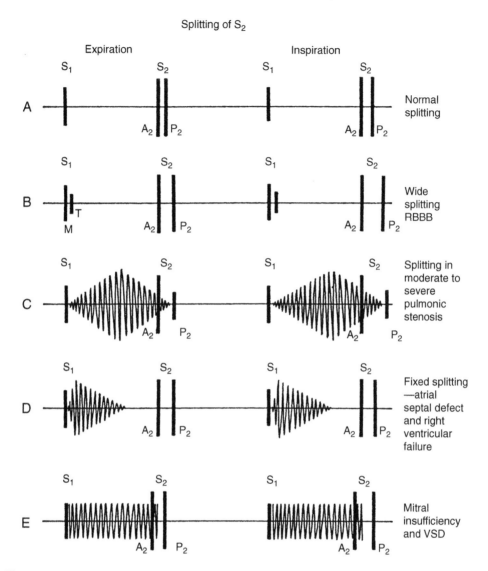

Figure 1-12 A, Normal splitting, audible only during inspiration. **B,** Wide splitting in right bundle-branch block (RBBB). Note the delayed P_2 during expiration, widening even more with inspiration. **C,** Wide splitting (pulmonic stenosis). Note the delayed P_2 during expiration, widening even more with inspiration. **D,** Fixed splitting (atrial septal defect and right ventricular failure). Note the delay of P_2 during expiration, uninfluenced by inspiration. **E,** Mitral insufficiency and ventricular septal defect (VSD). Note the early A_2, which is even more pronounced during inspiration. (*Modified from Leonard JJ, Kroetz RW, Shaver JA:* Examination of the heart: auscultation, *Dallas, 1974, American Heart Association.*)

✳ **KEY POINT** S_2 is heard best with the diaphragm at the left heart base.

As mentioned previously, the normal human ear differentiates, or can be trained to differentiate, between what are perceived as "crisp sounds" (single, brief sounds), "slurred" or "prolonged sounds" (either a slightly longer sound or two sounds separated by less than 0.02 second), and two distinct sounds (separated by at least 0.02 second). Thus splitting of S_2 is discernible only when A_2 and P_2 are separated by 0.02 second or more. Splitting is best appreciated with the diaphragm of the stethoscope.

Abnormal (pathologic, as opposed to physiologic) splitting of S_2 usually indicates a cardiovascular abnormality. The types of abnormal splitting include (1) persistent splitting, (2) "fixed" splitting, and (3) paradoxical splitting. Conditions causing wide splitting of S_2 with a normal A_2-P_2 relationship are listed in Box 1-4.

In persistent splitting, the A_2-P_2 interval is wider than normal throughout the respiratory cycle. The normal widening of the split during inspiration and narrowing with expiration still occur, but without expiratory fusion of S_2 into a single sound (see Figure 1-12).

In fixed splitting, the A_2-P_2 interval is also wider than normal throughout the respiratory cycle, but respiratory variation is minimal (less than 0.010 to 0.015 second, which is nearly imperceptible). The S_2 split sounds "fixed" or constant during both inspiration and expiration (see Figure 1-12).

In paradoxical splitting, aortic valve closure is significantly delayed with respect to pulmonic valve closure and the aortic valve may close after the pulmonic valve, reversing the normal sequence. P_2 now precedes A_2. The S_2 split actually increases during expiration (P_2 is earlier than A_2, and P_2 gets even earlier in expiration) and decreases with inspiration

---

■ **Box 1-4 Conditions Causing Wide Splitting of S_2**

Delayed Pulmonic Closure
Delayed right ventricular activation
  Right bundle-branch block
  Paced beats (left ventricular)
  Left ventricular ectopic beats
Prolonged right ventricular mechanical systole
  Pulmonic stenosis with intact ventricular septum (moderate to severe)
  Acute massive pulmonary embolus
  Pulmonary hypertension with right-sided heart failure
  Heartworm disease
Decreased impedance of the pulmonary vascular bed
  Atrial septal defect (normotensive)
  Pulmonary artery dilation (idiopathic)
  Pulmonic stenosis (mild)
Unexplained auditory expiratory splitting in an otherwise normal heart

Early Aortic Closure
Shortened left ventricular ejection time
  Mitral insufficiency
  Ventricular septal defect

From Shaver JA, O'Toole JD: The second heart sound: newer concepts. Part 1: normal and wide physiological splitting, *Mod Concepts Cardiovasc Dis* 46(2):7-12, 1977. By permission of the American Heart Association.

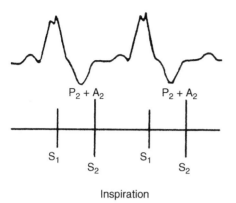

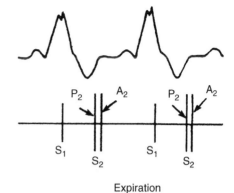

Inspiration

Expiration

Figure 1-13 **Paradoxical splitting of S$_2$ in a patient with left bundle-branch block (LBBB).**

■ **Box 1-5** Paradoxical Splitting of S$_2$

Left bundle-branch block
Right ventricular pacemaker
Patent ductus arteriosus
Aortic stenosis
Significant aortic regurgitation
Significant systemic hypertension

(because A$_2$ is before P$_2$, and P$_2$ is delayed with inspiration), resulting in paradoxical splitting (Figure 1-13). Conditions that may be associated with paradoxical splitting are listed in Box 1-5.

✳ **KEY POINT** A split and loud S$_2$ in dogs should prompt concern about pulmonary hypertension and possible heartworm disease.

The loudness of S$_2$ is determined by the sum of A$_2$ and P$_2$. An abnormally accentuated S$_2$ may be caused by augmentation of either component. Causes of abnormal accentuation of A$_2$ and P$_2$ are listed in Box 1-6. When P$_2$ is abnormally accentuated, it is significantly louder than A$_2$ in the pulmonic area. In dogs, pulmonary hypertension is probably the most commonly recognized cause of abnormally loud or "cracking" S$_2$. Conditions that may be associated with abnormal diminution of S$_2$ are listed in Box 1-7.

S$_2$ may not be audible or even present in some tachyarrhythmias. Depending on the timing and nature of the ectopic beat, ventricular filling may be inadequate to allow a contraction strong enough to cause opening and subsequent closing of the semilunar valves, creating a pulse deficit and an S$_1$ that is not followed by an audible S$_2$.

◀)) Third Heart Sound (S$_3$)

Blood flows quickly into the ventricle during the rapid filling phase of the cardiac cycle, early in diastole. In dogs and cats the normal ventricles can accommodate this blood

■ **Box 1-6** Abnormally Accentuated S$_2$

Abnormally Accentuated A$_2$
Systemic hypertension
Aortic dilation or aneurysm of ascending aorta
Valvular aortic stenosis (noncalcified valve)

Abnormally Accentuated P$_2$
Pulmonary hypertension secondary to congestive heart failure
Congenital left-to-right shunts
    Patent ductus arteriosus
    Ventricular septal defect
    Atrial septal defect
Primary pulmonary hypertension
Pulmonary embolism
Idiopathic dilation of the pulmonary artery
Mild valvular pulmonic stenosis
Heartworm disease

■ **Box 1-7** Abnormally Diminished S$_2$

Total Diminution of S$_2$ (Markedly Decreased Ventricular Function)
Hypothyroidism
Shock
Dilated cardiomyopathy

Diminished A$_2$
Significant calcific valvular aortic stenosis
Marked aortic regurgitation

Diminished P$_2$
Significant pulmonic stenosis of any cause

---

silently. If inflowing blood meets a ventricle that is less compliant than normal, however, the rapid deceleration of the ventricular wall and column of blood contained within the ventricle may result in audible, low-frequency vibrations that are known as the third heart sound (S$_3$; see Figure 1-7). S$_3$ is usually a left ventricular sound (the left ventricle is more massive and is prone to being less compliant) and is heard best at the left cardiac apex with the bell of the stethoscope applied lightly to the chest wall (Figure 1-14). In veterinary patients S$_3$ occurs most often under conditions of volume overload (e.g., dilated cardiomyopathy, long-standing and severe mitral insufficiency). Occasionally S$_3$ originates in the right ventricle and is best heard in the tricuspid area. Causes of S$_3$ are listed in Box 1-8.

✳ **KEY POINT** Third and fourth heart sounds are best heard with the bell of the stethoscope at the left cardiac apex.

S$_3$ may be accentuated by maneuvers that increase blood flow to the heart (e.g., exercise, excitement). Reduction of venous return by prolonged rest often reduces the intensity or even abolishes S$_3$. S$_3$ also shows characteristic respiratory variation in loudness, with the

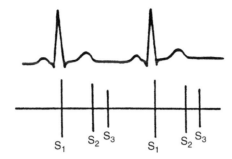

Figure 1-14 S_3 in a Doberman Pinscher with dilated cardiomyopathy.

■ **Box 1-8** Causes of S_3 Gallop

Left ventricular diastolic overload
   Mitral regurgitation
   Aortic regurgitation
   Left-to-right shunts
   High-output states
Right ventricular diastolic overload
   Tricuspid regurgitation
   Pulmonary regurgitation
   Left-to-right shunts
   High-output states
Diminished ventricular compliance or elevated ventricular mean diastolic pressure or both
   Cardiomyopathies
   Ventricular failure
   Ischemic heart disease

From Tilkian AG, Conover MB: *Understanding heart sounds and murmurs*, ed 4, Philadelphia, 2001, Saunders.

---

left ventricular S_3 accentuated during expiration and the occasional right ventricular S_3 augmented during inspiration. S_3 should be considered pathologic in dogs and cats until proved otherwise, although it is frequently a normal finding in animals with much more massive hearts (e.g., horses and cows). S_3 is often called a protodiastolic or ventricular gallop sound.

✳ **KEY POINT** The higher the inflow rate, the greater the rate of deceleration and the louder the resultant S_3. S_3 occurs often in conditions in which the ventricle is stiff and inflow is rapid, including some high-output states, mitral or tricuspid regurgitation, and dilated cardiomyopathy.

Fourth Heart Sound (S_4)

Like S_3, S_4 occurs during a phase of the cardiac cycle when the ventricle is expected to accept a large amount of blood quickly—in this case just after atrial contraction, immediately before ventricular systole (see Figure 1-7). The pathogenesis of S_4 is similar to S_3: an abnormally stiff (in the case of dogs and cats) ventricle decelerates abruptly and causes audible, low-frequency vibrations during what should be a rapid filling period. S_4 is also called an atrial gallop sound or a presystolic gallop. S_4 may be a right-sided or left-sided sound. A right-sided S_4 (from the right ventricle) is heard best in the tricuspid area and increases in loudness during inspiration. A left-sided S_4 (from the left ventricle) is auscultated best at the left cardiac apex and is augmented during expiration. Clinical observations in veterinary medicine suggest that S_4 gallops occur most often in animals with concentric left ventricular hypertrophy, such as hypertrophic cardiomyopathy. A presystolic (S_4) gallop is considered to indicate pathology in dogs and cats until proved otherwise. Cardiac conditions that may be associated with a right-sided or left-sided S_4 are listed in Box 1-9.

> ✳ **KEY POINT** Third and fourth heart sounds usually indicate pathology in dogs and cats.

S_4, like S_3, is a low-pitched heart sound (Figure 1-15). It is heard best with the bell of the stethoscope lightly applied to the chest wall. As with an S_3, the sound may be accentuated by increasing blood flow to the heart with exercise. Maneuvers reducing venous return diminish an S_4 or cause it to disappear.

Quadruple Rhythm, Summation Sounds, or Gallops

At times all four heart sounds may be heard, forming a so-called quadruple rhythm (Figure 1-16). When both S_3 and S_4 are present and the heart rate accelerates, as the time spent in diastole decreases, S_3 and S_4 approach each other and may be heard as a single sound known as a summation sound (SS) or summation gallop (Figure 1-17). Because of the high heart rates in cats, summation sounds are presumably more common in this species than in dogs.

▪ **Box 1-9** Causes of S_4 Gallop

Left ventricular systolic overload
    Systemic hypertension
    Left ventricular outflow obstruction
    Coarctation of the aorta
Right ventricular systolic overload
    Pulmonary hypertension
    Right ventricular outflow obstruction
    Pulmonary artery stenosis
Diminished ventricular compliance or elevated ventricular end-diastolic pressure or both
    Cardiomyopathies
    Ventricular failure
    Ischemic heart disease
    Myocardial infarction
Other causes associated with augmented ventricular filling
    Thyrotoxicosis
    Anemia
    Mitral regurgitation (acute, severe)
    Large arteriovenous fistulae
Complete heart block (S_4 occurs randomly in diastole)

From Tilkian AG, Conover MB: *Understanding heart sounds and murmurs*, ed 4, Philadelphia, 2001, Saunders.

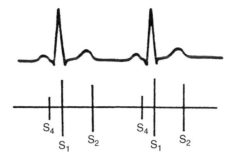

Figure 1-15 S_4 in a cat with hypertrophic cardiomyopathy.

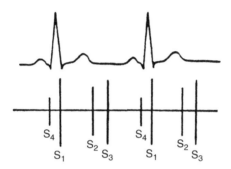

Figure 1-16 A quadruple rhythm formed by S_1, S_2, S_3, and S_4.

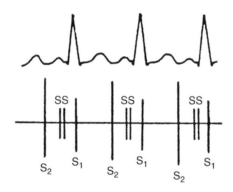

Figure 1-17 A summation sound (SS) formed by S_3 and S_4 in a cat with dilated cardiomyopathy.

KEY POINT S_3 gallop is most commonly auscultated in dogs with volume overloads, as seen with mitral valve disease and dilated cardiomyopathy. S_4 gallops are most commonly heard in cats with hypertrophic cardiomyopathy.

Ejection Sounds or Clicks

Ejection sounds or clicks (ESs) are discrete, high-frequency sounds following the first main component of S_1 (M_1) and occurring at the time of onset of ventricular ejection (Figure 1-18). ESs may arise from either the aortic or pulmonic circulation. The terms "ejection

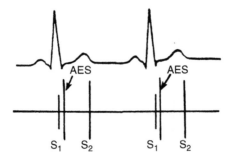

Figure 1-18 Aortic ejection sounds (AESs) in a patient with aortic valve stenosis.

■ **Box 1-10** Aortic Ejection Sounds

Associated with forceful left ventricular ejection
  Hyperthyroidism
  Exercise
  Anemia
  Other high-output states
Dilation of the ascending aorta with or without systemic hypertension
Valvular aortic stenosis

---

sound" and "ejection click" are frequently used interchangeably, depending on the quality of the sound. When the sound is very high pitched, brief, and "clicky," it is called an ejection click. When the "clicky" quality is absent, it is often referred to as an ejection sound. Ejection sounds or clicks are uncommon in dogs and cats.

Aortic ejection sounds (AESs) are heard best at the left heart base. AESs appear to have two causes. The first type of AES results from energy release and vibrations with onset of ejection of blood from the left ventricle into the aorta and may represent accentuation of the normal second main component of S_1. This AES may occur with increased or forceful flow into the aorta or with systemic hypertension and is often associated with aortic root dilation. The second type of AES occurs in valvular aortic stenosis (a rare condition in dogs and cats) as the abnormally fused aortic valve reaches the limit of its opening just after the start of ventricular ejection.

Because AESs are high-pitched sounds, they are heard best with the diaphragm of the stethoscope. Recognition of an AES during auscultation depends on the relative loudness of S_1 and AES and the interval separating the sounds. The sound combination should be differentiated from an S_4-S_1 or split S_1 combination. The high pitch of ESs helps differentiate them from the low-pitched S_4. Box 1-10 lists clinical conditions that may be accompanied by an AES.

Pulmonic ejection sounds (PESs) are auscultated best in the pulmonic area and along the left sternal border. PESs follow M_1 (Figure 1-19). PESs may be associated with valvular pulmonic stenosis (which is far more common than valvular aortic stenosis) or may arise from the pulmonary artery with or without pulmonary hypertension. PESs occur with the onset of ejection of blood from the right ventricle into the pulmonary artery. The PESs with valvular pulmonic stenosis typically occur earlier in systole and in our experience are

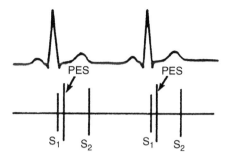

Figure 1-19 Pulmonic ejection sounds (PESs) in a patient with pulmonic valve stenosis.

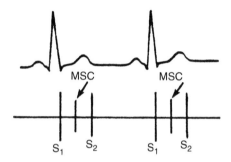

Figure 1-20 Midsystolic clicks (MSCs) in an animal with mitral valve prolapse.

Box 1-11 Pulmonic Ejection Sounds

Dilated main pulmonary artery with pulmonary hypertension
    Heartworm disease
    Recurrent pulmonary emboli
    Primary pulmonary hypertension
Dilated main pulmonary artery without pulmonary hypertension
    Idiopathic dilatation of pulmonary artery
    Atrial septal defect
Valvular pulmonic stenosis

most often confused with an extremely loud S_1. PESs are also heard best with the diaphragm of the stethoscope. Cardiac conditions that may be associated with a PES are listed in Box 1-11.

Midsystolic Click or Clicks

Midsystolic clicks (MSCs) are discrete, high-frequency sounds that usually occur during mid- to late-ventricular systole (Figure 1-20). These sounds are best heard with the diaphragm of the stethoscope over the mitral and tricuspid valve areas. MSCs may be present alone, may initiate or occur during midsystolic to late-systolic murmurs, or may occur in the presence of or be obscured by a holosystolic murmur. Lability of timing and intensity characterizes the MSC, which at any given time may be absent, single, or multiple and may be either midsystolic or late systolic in occurrence. In humans most MSCs are attributed to sudden tension of redundant chordae tendineae or leaflets of the mitral valve when abnormal mitral valve prolapse occurs during ventricular systole. They are heard occasionally in dogs with myxomatous degeneration of the mitral valve. Systolic clicks have also been noted as incidental findings in dogs without apparent cardiac disease, but in Cavalier King Charles Spaniels they are often associated with mitral valve prolapse and are considered by many to be the harbingers of future chronic valvular heart disease.

● Posttest 1

Part A

1. Left bundle-branch block can cause paradoxical splitting of S_2.
   a. True
   b. False

2. Ejection sounds are common in cats and dogs.
   a. True
   b. False

3. S_2 is louder in patients with severe pulmonic stenosis.
   a. True
   b. False

4. The left ventricular S_3 is heard best at the left apex.
   a. True
   b. False

5. During inspiration, blood flow to the right ventricle is increased.
   a. True
   b. False

6. Persistent splitting of S_2 can be seen with canine heartworm disease.
   a. True
   b. False

7. S_3 is a lower pitched heart sound than S_2.
   a. True
   b. False

8. Summation gallops are presumably less common in cats than dogs because of the higher heart rates in cats.
   a. True
   b. False

9. S_3 is considered normal in puppies and kittens.
   a. True
   b. False

10. S_3 is a low-frequency sound that is heard best with the bell of the stethoscope.
    a. True
    b. False

Part B

Directions: *Part B consists of 10 unknowns presented on the accompanying website. After determining the correct answers, fill in the appropriate blanks. Pay close attention to the location and timing of the heart sounds. Because you are not examining the patient, the location and, where appropriate, the timing are provided.*

 1. Apex. _____

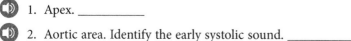 2. Aortic area. Identify the early systolic sound. _____

3. Apex. Identify the diastolic sound. If the rate were lower, two diastolic sounds would be heard. _____

4. Pulmonic area. _____

5. Apex. Identify the sound following S_2. _____

6. Apex. Identify the midsystolic sounds. _____

7. Pulmonic area. Identify the early systolic sound. _____

8. Apex. Identify the sound preceding S_1. _____

9. Pulmonic area. This Great Dane has a normal ECG. _____

10. Pulmonic area. _____

Murmurs

Objectives

Upon completion of this program, you should be able to:

1. List the steps to be employed to evaluate heart murmurs properly.
2. Explain the grading of murmurs.
3. Explain, on the basis of frequency (i.e., cps, Hz), shape, and timing, the various types of systolic and diastolic murmurs.
4. State the characteristics of the murmur of aortic stenosis.
5. List the auscultatory findings associated with ventricular septal defects.
6. List criteria that are useful in differentiating innocent or physiologic from pathologic murmurs.
7. Recognize the auscultatory findings of mitral regurgitation.
8. Explain the origin of the systolic murmur of atrial septal defect.
9. State the effect of respiration on the murmur of tricuspid regurgitation.
10. Recognize the murmur of patent ductus arteriosus.

• Pretest 2

1. A palpable vibration on the chest wall sometimes accompanies a loud heart murmur. If the murmur producing the vibration cannot be heard without placing the stethoscope on the chest wall, the grade of the murmur would be described as

   _____.
   a. II/VI
   b. III/VI
   c. IV/VI
   d. V/VI

2. The point of maximal intensity of the murmur of a small perimembranous ventricular septal defect is usually the _____.
   a. right sternal border
   b. left apex
   c. right heart base
   d. carotid artery

3. Crescendo-decrescendo murmurs are characteristic of _____.
   a. mitral valve regurgitation
   b. subaortic stenosis
   c. aortic valve regurgitation
   d. tricuspid valve regurgitation

4. Which of the following characteristics are often true of physiologic (Still's or flow) murmurs?
   a. They are often heard best at the left heart base.
   b. They are often soft murmurs (grade I or II/VI).
   c. They most often occur in young animals, less than a year of age.
   d. All of the above are true.

5. Which of the following murmur descriptions is accurate?
   a. The murmur is caused by a small atrial septal defect and is often diastolic.
   b. The murmur is caused by aortic valve regurgitation, is diastolic, and is loudest at the left heart base.
   c. The murmur of pulmonary valve stenosis is systolic and usually heard best on the right side of the chest
   d. For equal volumes of blood regurgitated, the murmur of tricuspid regurgitation will be louder than the murmur of mitral regurgitation.

6. Aortic valve endocarditis often occurs in the setting of underlying subaortic stenosis. If the infection causes the valve to leak, this combination of defects will cause a

   _____.
   a. systolic murmur, loudest at the right apex
   b. systolic murmur, loudest at the right heart base
   c. a "to and fro" murmur, loudest at the left heart base
   d. a musical murmur at the left apex

7. Early in the course of the disease, mitral valve endocardiosis may cause which of the following auscultatory findings?
   a. Soft S_3 gallop
   b. Systolic click
   c. Systolic murmur loudest at the left apex
   d. Both b and c are correct.

8. Which of the following statements about the murmur of tricuspid regurgitation is true?
   a. It may be heard in conjunction with the louder murmur of mitral regurgitation, making it difficult to know if the mitral murmur is radiating to the right side or whether tricuspid regurgitation is present.
   b. It may increase in intensity when pulmonary hypertension develops.
   c. It may increase in intensity with the intake of a deep breath.
   d. All of the above statements are true.

9. The murmur in ventricular septal defect is caused by blood flow across the defect from the left ventricle to the right ventricle. Which of the following is true?
   a. The murmur of a VSD would be expected to increase in intensity with the presence of systemic hypertension.
   b. The murmur of a VSD would be expected to decrease in intensity with the presence of pulmonary hypertension.
   c. Concurrent polycythemia (increased red cell mass or PCV) would be expected to decrease the intensity of a VSD murmur.
   d. All of the above statements are true.

10. In cats _____.
   a. murmurs of both dynamic outflow tract obstruction and mitral valve regurgitation are sometimes heard best at the left sternal border
   b. the murmur of an isolated VSD is best heard at the right sternal border
   c. heart rates in excess of 240 beats/minute can make assessing the timing of transient heart sounds and murmurs more difficult
   d. All of the above

Abbreviations

A_2	Aortic component of S_2	**PMI**	Point of maximal intensity
ASD	Atrial septal defect	S_1	First heart sound
AV	Atrioventricular	S_2	Second heart sound
cps	Cycles per second	S_3	Third heart sound
Hz	Hertz (cycles per second, a	S_4	Fourth heart sound
	synonym of cps above)	**SAM**	Systolic anterior motion of the
ICS	Intercostal space		mitral valve
P_2	Pulmonic component of S_2	T_1	Second main component of S_1
PDA	Patent ductus arteriosus	**VSD**	Ventricular septal defect

Evaluation of Heart Murmurs

Heart murmurs are prolonged sounds, generally caused by turbulent blood flow within the heart or great vessels. Whether or not turbulence forms depends on several physiologic factors, including the velocity of the blood flow, the size of the chamber or vessel receiving the blood flow, and the viscosity of the blood (which under normal circumstances depends mostly on the packed cell volume). The relationship between these variables and the formation of turbulence is described by Reynolds number, and the tendency for flow to become turbulent increases with increasing blood flow velocity and chamber size and decreases with increasing blood viscosity.

Murmurs often radiate or travel in the direction of turbulent blood flow (e.g., the murmur of aortic stenosis is heard best at the left heart base, over the aortic valve, but it is also heard well at the right heart base, because the aortic arch normally crosses to the right hemithorax high up under the right foreleg of the dog and cat, at the right heart base). In addition to the direction of blood flow, the efficiency of the acoustic coupling of the cardiovascular structure(s) generating the sound to the chest wall at a particular location may play an important role in where the sound is heard on the chest. A description of a murmur should include its anatomic location (point of maximal intensity [PMI]), radiation, timing (when it occurs in the cardiac cycle), intensity (loudness), pitch (frequency), and quality (the "shape" of the murmur when recorded on paper by a phonocardiograph).

The examiner can generally adequately describe location by noting the side of the chest on which the murmur seems loudest, as well as whether it is loudest at the cardiac apex, base, or some other location (e.g., right sternal border at the level of the cardiac apex). The location(s) to which a murmur radiates (see discussion of intensity, below) should also be noted. Although murmurs in dogs can often be localized to the affected valve area or area of turbulent flow, most murmurs in cats have a sternal or parasternal location.

✳ **KEY POINT** Murmurs in cats often have a sternal location.

Timing is determined by the period of the cardiac cycle during which the turbulent blood flow responsible for the murmur develops. Timing should be noted to be systolic (between S_1 and S_2; modifications might include "early," "mid," or "late," which are self-explanatory, or "holo," meaning throughout systole, depending on when the murmur was heard during systole), diastolic (between S_2 and S_1; the same modifiers can be applied), both systolic and diastolic (two separate murmurs with a quiet period between systole and diastole, such as the "to-and-fro" murmur of aortic stenosis and aortic regurgitation), or continuous (one murmur, most commonly caused by patent ductus arteriosus [PDA], which often peaks around S_2; there is no quiet period that separates the sound). Systolic murmurs are the murmurs most commonly found in dogs and cats. Common causes include atrioventricular (AV) valve insufficiency (mitral insufficiency or regurgitation is the most common) and semilunar valve stenosis. Diastolic murmurs are far less common in dogs, the most frequent clinical example being aortic insufficiency associated with aortic valve endocarditis. Diastolic murmurs are extremely rare in cats. Murmurs that are both systolic and diastolic in timing are unusual and often described as "to-and-fro" murmurs. The most common example of a to-and-fro murmur is the combination of aortic stenosis and aortic insufficiency (often associated with endocarditis or congenital heart disease). Continuous murmurs are most frequently caused by congenital PDA, although other causes, including arteriovenous fistula, ruptured coronary artery–right atrial aneurysm, and aorticopulmonary window with left-to-right shunting, are occasionally found.

✳ **KEY POINT** The most common murmurs are systolic and caused by AV valve insufficiency or semilunar valve stenosis.

Intensity, or loudness, of heart murmurs is graded on a semisubjective scale from I to VI. The grades provide a means by which clinicians can communicate with one another regarding the intensity of murmurs, and although the grading system is not universally accepted, they are defined here as follows:

- I/VI signifies a very soft murmur heard only in a quiet room after a period of concentrated listening over the point on the chest where the murmur is heard.
- II/VI is a soft murmur that is audible as soon as the stethoscope chestpiece is appropriately placed at the PMI. A II/VI murmur does not radiate widely from the point on the chest where it is heard best.
- III/VI is louder, heard easily some distance away from its PMI (but not generally audible on the opposite side of the chest).
- IV/VI signifies a loud murmur, radiating widely (often including the opposite side of the chest), but not associated with a palpable precordial thrill.
- V/VI designates a very loud murmur associated with a palpable precordial thrill that always marks its PMI on the chest wall.
- VI/VI designates an extremely loud murmur that not only is associated with a palpable precordial thrill, but also can be heard without the stethoscope or with the stethoscope removed from the chest wall.

Pitch describes the auscultator's perception of the frequency of the murmur, and because of the inexactness of most people's ears as a gauge of pitch (the ability to accurately assess frequency, known as perfect pitch, is a relatively rare gift among humans), comments are often limited to "high-" (>300 Hz), "mid-" (100-300 Hz), or "low-" (<100 Hz) pitched murmurs. Occasionally murmurs are described as "musical" (containing a pure tone, often heard as a literal "buzz," rather than a mixture of frequencies that sound like a harsh "shhhhhh"), and low-frequency murmurs are often perceived as "rumbles."

Quality, or shape, of a murmur is most often described as ejection (crescendo-decrescendo or diamond shaped), regurgitant (also called plateau shaped or rectangular),

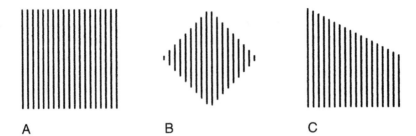

A   B   C

Figure 2-1 Common configurations of cardiac murmurs. A, Plateau. B, Crescendo-decrescendo. C, Decrescendo.

▪ Table 2-1 Breed Predilections for Cardiac Disorders

Disorder	Breed Predilection
Aortic stenosis	Boxer, German Shepherd, Golden Retriever, Newfoundland, Rottweiler
Atrial septal defect	Samoyed, Standard Poodle
Mitral valve dysplasia	Chihuahua, English Bulldog, Great Dane, Newfoundland
Patent ductus arteriosus	Collie, German Shepherd, Irish Setter, Pomeranian, Poodle, Shetland Sheepdog, Corgi
Pulmonic stenosis	Beagle, Chihuahua, English Bulldog, Schnauzer, Terriers
Tetralogy of Fallot	Keeshond, English Bulldog
Tricuspid valve dysplasia	Labrador Retriever, Weimaraner
Ventricular septal defect	English Springer Spaniel
Degenerative atrioventricular valve disease	Small-breed dogs, Cavalier King Charles Spaniel, Dachshund
Dilated cardiomyopathy	Large- and giant-breed dogs, Doberman Pinscher, Boxer, Portuguese Water Spaniel
Hypertrophic cardiomyopathy	Maine Coon, Ragdoll, Sphinx, British Shorthair, Persian

blowing (decrescendo), or machinery (synonymous with continuous; machinery murmurs often peak in intensity around S_2) (Figure 2-1).

Knowledge of the timing and location of a murmur allows the practitioner to establish a differential diagnosis rapidly (Figure 2-2). The differential diagnosis can often be narrowed further by consideration of the signalment (species, age, breed, and gender) and intensity. This is especially true for congenital heart defects (Table 2-1). Systolic murmurs developing in mature small-breed dogs are typically caused by progression of chronic mitral or mitral and tricuspid valve disease (endocardiosis). Acquired soft systolic murmurs in large- or giant-breed dogs are often caused by dilated cardiomyopathy. The likely cause of an acquired murmur in cats varies with the cat's age. Hypertrophic cardiomyopathy is the most common cause in young and middle-aged cats. Systemic hypertension, hyperthyroidism, and valvular disease are more common in senior cats.

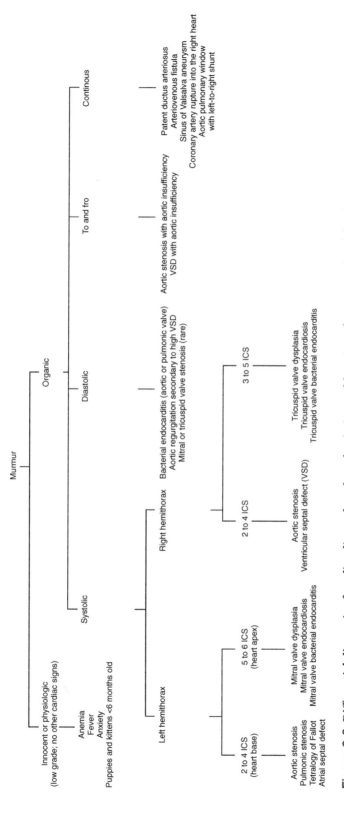

Figure 2-2 Differential diagnosis of cardiac disease based on the timing and location of murmurs. *(Modified from Allen DG: Murmurs and abnormal heart sounds. In Allen DG, Kruth SA, editors: Small animal cardiopulmonary medicine, Philadelphia, 1988, BC Decker.)*

Turbulent blood flow leading to heart murmurs can result from two main factors: (1) high-velocity blood flow (e.g., the heart pumps a greater than normal volume of blood through a normal valve opening with each beat, or a normal volume of blood is forced through a narrowed [stenotic] valve) or (2) normal-velocity blood flow but low-viscosity blood (i.e., turbulence forms at a normal flow velocity because of reduced blood viscosity, usually caused by anemia). Blood flow velocities high enough to generate audible turbulence through normal valves can occur when blood is shunted from one side of the heart to another under low pressure, resulting in a volume overload (e.g., in atrial septal defect [ASD] where the pressure difference between the left and right atrium is small, such that the velocity of blood flowing from the left to the right atrium is low and no turbulence forms despite a potentially large volume of blood being shunted from the left to the right atrium). The murmur in ASDs is caused by the turbulent flow of that larger than normal amount of blood across the normal pulmonic valve, which is generally much smaller in diameter than either the ASD or the tricuspid valve. Conditions in which the cardiac output is elevated (e.g., exercise, excitement, fever, hyperthyroidism) may also cause audible turbulent blood flow to form across normal valves. Generally, a murmur caused by the mechanism of increased blood flowing across normal heart valves is a relatively low-intensity (soft) murmur. Otherwise normal cats sometimes develop relatively mild dynamic right ventricular outflow tract obstruction (the dynamic contraction of the right ventricular outflow tract narrows it, accelerating blood flow sufficiently to cause turbulence), resulting in a heart murmur. Flow of normal quantities of blood across narrowed (stenotic) valves can also result in elevations of blood flow velocity sufficient to cause audible turbulence to form. This mechanism can often produce intense (loud) murmurs, and the intensity of such murmurs is generally directly related to the severity of the stenosis (which determines the flow velocity) as long as the cardiac output and blood viscosity remain normal. Backward (regurgitant) blood flow through an incompetent valve or blood flow between two chambers with a high pressure differential that are not normally connected (e.g., ventricular septal defect [VSD] or PDA) also causes blood flow velocities high enough to generate audible turbulence and thus a murmur. Various combinations of these factors may be present and determine the timing, duration, shape, pitch, and loudness of the murmur.

Systolic Murmurs

Systolic murmurs are auscultated and recorded between S_1 and S_2, during the phases of left or right ventricular systole. Systolic murmurs may be divided into two main groups:

1. Ejection murmurs
2. Regurgitant murmurs

Systolic Ejection Murmurs

Systolic ejection murmurs start shortly after (not covering up) S_1, increase to a peak loudness in early, mid, or sometimes even late systole, and then decrease in loudness and terminate before S_2 (such that S_2 can also be heard in the presence of a systolic ejection murmur). These murmurs are caused by turbulent flow formation in the aorta or pulmonary artery during the ejection phase of systole, and the murmur thus generated is diamond shaped or crescendo-decrescendo, the shape of the sound reflecting the shape of the

■ **Box 2-1** Causes of Systolic Ejection Murmurs

Left ventricular outflow obstruction
    Discrete subaortic stenosis
    Valvular aortic stenosis
    Hypertrophic cardiomyopathy and other causes of left ventricular hypertrophy
    Systolic anterior motion of the mitral valve
Right ventricular outflow tract obstruction
    Valvular pulmonic stenosis
    Infundibular pulmonic stenosis/pulmonic valve dysplasia
    Tetralogy of Fallot
    Dynamic right ventricular outflow obstruction in cats
Hyperkinetic or high-flow states
    Congenital left-to-right shunt (e.g., atrial septal defect)
    Anemia
    Thyrotoxicosis
Functional (or innocent) systolic murmurs
Miscellaneous
    Dilation of aorta or pulmonary artery distal to semilunar valves

velocity profile of blood flow into the great vessel and the pressure gradient that generated it. Causes of systolic ejection murmurs are listed in Box 2-1.

Significant lesions in the first two categories of Box 2-1 (outflow tract stenoses) are typically associated with loud (grades III to VI), harsh systolic murmurs. Such murmurs are best characterized with the diaphragm of the stethoscope for clearest delineation of the main components of S_1 and S_2 and the dominant medium (with some high) frequencies of the systolic crescendo-decrescendo murmur.

Murmurs occurring with minimal or absent outflow tract obstruction, or the last three categories in Box 2-1, are typically shorter in duration, softer (grades I to II), and often heard best or only in the first third to half of systole. These murmurs have dominant medium (with some low) frequencies and are sometimes heard best with the bell of the stethoscope. Physiologic or Still's murmurs are thought to reflect the relatively small size of the aorta or pulmonary artery in relation to the relatively high cardiac output of some young (generally less than a year old) animals in the absence of an identifiable pathology. Some of these murmurs may in fact be associated with moderator bands or other ventricular structures that influence ventricular outflow. These murmurs sometimes have a musical component that is unusual in other ejection murmurs and that may change in intensity or duration with changes in the animal's body position. Several characteristic systolic ejection murmurs are described here.

✳ **KEY POINT** Physiologic murmurs in cats are common, accounting for 20% to 25% of murmurs.

Valvular aortic stenosis, when hemodynamically significant, reflects pathologic narrowing of the aortic valve to less than 50% of its normal area. This is a rare congenital defect in dogs and cats and is not discussed further here.

The systolic murmur of *subaortic stenosis* (also called subvalvular aortic stenosis) results from high-velocity blood flow across a left ventricular outflow tract obstruction located below the aortic valve. This is the most common form of aortic stenosis in dogs, constituting greater than 90% of all cases in most geographic (and therefore genetic) regions (Boxer dogs with ejection murmurs from "small aortas" represent an exception). The murmur is usually heard loudest in the aortic area and frequently radiates to the right hemithorax (around the second or third intercostal space [ICS]). The murmur may radiate up the carotid arteries and rarely to the calvarium. It is also a harsh or rough, medium- to high-pitched murmur, frequently of relatively long duration. As with valvular aortic stenosis, as a general rule the more severe the obstruction, the louder the murmur. Unlike valvular aortic stenosis in humans, the left ventricular outflow obstruction of subvalvular aortic stenosis in dogs may have a labile component because of additional subvalvular muscular impingement on the outflow tract. In such patients the loudness and duration of the murmur may vary significantly from examination to examination, with changes determined by the hemodynamic state of the patient.

> ✳ **KEY POINT** The murmur of aortic stenosis can markedly vary in loudness and may not be present in the first few months after birth.

Auscultatory clues in significant subaortic stenosis are as follows:

- Harsh, medium-pitched, loud (grade III or greater), long systolic ejection murmur with crescendo-decrescendo pattern (Figure 2-3).
- Murmur typically loudest in the aortic area and radiating to the area of the right thoracic inlet (the murmur may be nearly equally loud on the left and right heart base); murmur may radiate up the carotid arteries and rarely to the calvarium.
- Generally normal intensity S_1.
- Aortic ejection sound rarely heard (Figure 2-4).
- Variation in loudness and duration of the systolic murmur from examination to examination possible (particularly with labile obstruction).
- Murmur not always present from birth; may develop or become progressively louder over the first year of life.

Auscultatory findings similar to aortic stenosis may be present in cats with *hypertrophic cardiomyopathy* and *aortic outflow obstruction* caused by systolic anterior motion of the mitral valve (SAM). The murmur is usually loudest at the left sternal border or over the sternum and varies in loudness with heart rate (i.e., louder at higher rates) (Figure 2-5). It

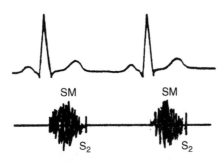

Figure 2-3 Crescendo-decrescendo systolic murmur (SM) of subaortic stenosis.

should be emphasized that not all cats with hypertrophic cardiomyopathy have aortic outflow obstruction. Cats with hypertrophic cardiomyopathy may also have regurgitant murmurs in the mitral valve area caused by SAM, papillary muscle dysfunction, or distortion of the mitral valve annulus from concentric hypertrophy.

The systolic murmur of significant *valvular pulmonic stenosis* (with intact ventricular septum) is similar in quality to the murmur of valvular aortic stenosis (harsh or rough, medium-pitched crescendo-decrescendo). The loudness and duration of the murmur are also closely and directly related to the severity of the stenosis. The murmur is usually well localized with maximal loudness in the pulmonic area and, unlike subaortic stenosis, is always clearly louder on the left side of the chest (although the patient may have a loud concurrent systolic regurgitant murmur on the right hemithorax associated with tricuspid valve insufficiency, a common secondary problem in severe pulmonic stenosis). Even when the stenosis is mild, abnormal splitting of S_2 (persistent splitting with an increased A_2-P_2 interval) is usually present, although this is difficult to appreciate without a phonocardiogram. Splitting may be difficult to hear owing to the decreased intensity of P_2 and the murmur.

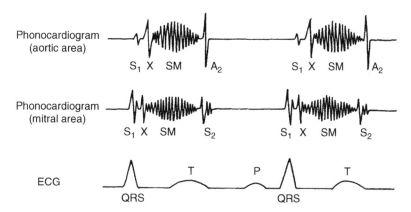

Figure 2-4 **Ejection sound (X) of congenital aortic stenosis.** Note that this sound is louder in the aortic area than it is in the mitral area. *SM,* Systolic murmur. *(From Tilkian AG, Conover MB:* Understanding heart sounds and murmurs, *ed 4, Philadelphia, 2001, Saunders.)*

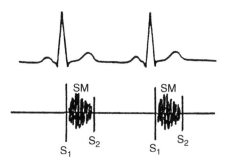

Figure 2-5 **Systolic ejection murmur (SM) in a cat with hypertrophic cardiomyopathy.**

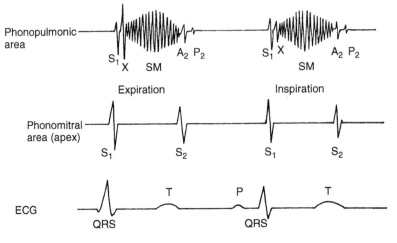

Figure 2-6 Ejection sound (X) of pulmonic stenosis. Note that this sound is not heard in the mitral area and that it significantly decreases during inspiration. Note also the diminished P₂ in the presence of pulmonic stenosis. *SM,* Systolic murmur. *(From Tilkian AG, Conover MB: Understanding heart sounds and murmurs, ed 4, Philadelphia, 2001, Saunders.)*

✳ **KEY POINT** It is important not to miss the murmur of pulmonic stenosis or PDA, because these defects can be corrected.

Auscultatory clues in significant valvular pulmonic stenosis are as follows:

- Harsh, medium-pitched to high-pitched, loud (grade III or greater), long systolic ejection murmur (Figure 2-6).
- Systolic murmur loudest in the pulmonic area (left heart base) with wide radiation.
- Relatively normal S₁.
- May be associated with an opening "snap," a sound that occurs when the fused valve leaflets reach their opening limit. This sometimes loud sound may be heard as an early systolic click or is sometimes confused with a loud or split S₁.
- Abnormally wide splitting of S₂ (usually difficult to appreciate).
- P₂ may appear diminished in severe stenosis with a loud murmur, but S₂ is audible.

The murmur associated with *tetralogy of Fallot* is variable and complex owing to the presence of multiple defects of variable severity. Murmurs include a right sternal border murmur associated with the VSD and a left basilar murmur associated with the pulmonic stenosis. The pulmonic ejection murmur tends to predominate. The nature and intensity of the murmur reflect the severity of the aortic override (and subsequent pulmonic stenosis or hypoplasia), as well as the degree of subsequent right-to-left shunting. Mild pulmonic obstruction with minimal aortic malposition may be associated with subsystemic right ventricular pressures, absence of cyanosis and attendant polycythemia, and presence of a loud holosystolic murmur at the right sternal border. More severe aortic override and pulmonic stenosis or hypoplasia cause right ventricular pressures to become supersystemic, with subsequent right-to-left shunting of blood through the VSD and the development of cyanosis and polycythemia. Animals with this constellation of anatomic structures (dogs

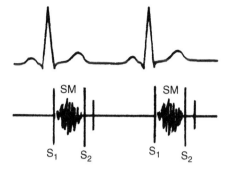

Figure 2-7 Atrial septal defect. The systolic ejection murmur (SM) is followed by fixed splitting of S_2.

and cats) tend to have relatively soft systolic ejection murmurs (for their degree of obstruction), usually heard best at the left heart base.

The systolic murmur of *atrial septal defect* is characteristic of systolic murmurs present in hyperkinetic or high-flow states, as mentioned earlier. The murmur is crescendo-decrescendo in contour, usually medium pitched, and typically of short duration, ending well before the beginning of S_2. The murmur is generally most prominent in the pulmonic area. The murmur of ASD is not caused by blood flow across the defect; it is secondary to increased flow across the pulmonic valve and subsequent dilatation of the pulmonary artery. Small defects (and patent oval foramen) will not have an associated murmur.

Auscultatory clues in significant ASD are as follows:

- Medium-pitched, short systolic murmur with characteristic diamond-shaped contour, usually soft (grade I to II), occasionally grade III in loudness, heard best at the left heart base (Figure 2-7).
- Active right precordium associated with right ventricular and atrial volume loading in significant defects.
- Frequent accentuation of S_1 in the tricuspid valve region (owing to accentuation of the T_1, a component of S_1).
- Abnormally wide splitting of S_2, with "fixed" splitting (no movement of the split) during respiration. This is difficult to appreciate in animals, because respiratory movements are difficult to influence reliably.

Dynamic right ventricular obstruction is a recently reported cause of systolic murmurs originating in the right ventricular outflow tract of cats. The murmur is parasternal in location and is usually seen in cats older than 4 years of age. The murmur is usually associated with high-output states (e.g., inflammatory disease, hyperthyroidism, anemia) and chronic renal failure with or without systemic hypertension. Cats with this murmur younger than 4 years of age often have concurrent cardiac disease. *Dynamic left ventricular outflow obstruction* also occurs commonly in cats, often as a result of systolic anterior motion of the mitral valve, as mentioned following the discussion of aortic stenosis. Dynamic sub-aortic stenosis can also occur with volume depletion and left ventricular hypertrophy.

✳ **KEY POINT** Systolic murmurs in cats are often associated with dynamic right or left ventricular outflow obstruction.

Murmurs associated purely with anemia are usually not detected until the hemoglobin level drops below 6 mg/dL, usually corresponding to a hematocrit of less than 18%. The murmur is caused by decreased blood viscosity and the subsequent formation of turbulence—the guideline of a hematocrit of less than 18% to achieve reductions in blood viscosity is just that, because other factors may affect viscosity. The murmur associated with anemia is soft (grade III or less) and occurs during early systole to midsystole. The murmur is usually heard best at the left heart base. It is worth remembering that in addition to causing murmurs when severe, anemia can increase the intensity of otherwise inaudible or soft murmurs caused by potentially minor cardiac defects.

Innocent systolic murmurs are also called functional, physiologic, or Still's murmurs (murmurs not associated with any organic heart disease, as mentioned previously). These systolic ejection murmurs may be heard in normal animals of all ages but are found mainly in puppies and kittens less than a year of age. The murmurs emanate, at least partly, from turbulence in the aortic root or pulmonary artery caused by forward flow across the normal left or right ventricular outflow tracts.

Auscultatory clues in innocent systolic murmurs are as follows:

- Usually soft (grade I to II) systolic murmur of short duration in early systole (Figure 2-8).
- S_1 and S_2 normal.
- Absence of abnormal sounds (e.g., ejection sounds, S_3 or S_4) or diastolic murmurs.
- May be musical.
- May change in intensity or disappear with changes in body position during auscultation.

Holosystolic or Regurgitant Murmurs

Holosystolic murmurs are typically characterized by (1) longer duration than systolic ejection murmurs, with murmurs beginning with S_1 and ending with or actually enveloping and obscuring S_2; (2) a plateau or rectangular configuration with relatively uniform loudness throughout systole; and (3) dominant high frequencies with less harsh or rough quality to the murmur than is commonly found with ejection quality murmurs.

The typical holosystolic murmur is best initially auscultated with the diaphragm of the stethoscope. Murmurs that are caused by AV valve regurgitation may in fact be less than holosystolic and may have varying configurations, durations, and frequencies owing to the

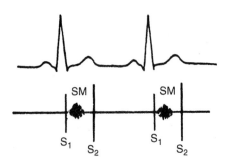

🔊 Figure 2-8 Innocent low-intensity systolic ejection murmur (SM) in an asymptomatic puppy.

anatomic and pathophysiologic features responsible for the leaky valve. Causes of holosystolic murmurs are listed below. Generally, regurgitant quality murmurs occur when two chambers that have dramatically different pressures throughout systole experience an abnormal connection during this time (e.g., a VSD permitting high-velocity blood flow from the high-pressure left ventricle into the low-pressure right ventricle). The size of the hole is not necessarily related to the intensity of the murmur in such cases, because a small hole might be associated with severely turbulent flow.

Causes of holosystolic murmur include mitral regurgitation, tricuspid regurgitation, and VSD.

✳ **KEY POINT** The severity of the cardiac disorder is not always correlated with the loudness of the murmur.

Mitral Regurgitation

Coaptation (closure) of the mitral valve during systole depends on the complex interactions and coordination of the mitral annulus, the mitral valve leaflets, the chordae tendineae, and the papillary muscles. Malfunction of any of the components of this "mitral complex" can result in an abnormal regurgitant flow (leakage) of blood from the high-pressure left ventricle to the low-pressure left atrium during ventricular systole. Such regurgitant flow is nearly always turbulent because of its high velocity (driven by the large, relatively constant pressure differential between the ventricle and atrium during systole), and it is associated with a plateau-shaped heart murmur that reflects this constant pressure differential. The most common causes of mitral regurgitation are myxomatous degeneration of the mitral valve (which may progress to actual ruptured chordae tendineae), systemic hypertension, and cardiomyopathy.

Myxomatous Degeneration of the Mitral Valve. This defect is typically associated with a mitral regurgitant murmur that is usually heard throughout the period of systole (holosystolic). One or more systolic or nonejection clicks (see discussion of midsystolic clicks) may be auscultated if the mitral valve is prolapsing (actually moving or "tenting" beyond the normal closed position, such that part of the valve buckles back into the atrium). These clicks may precede the onset of the murmur and may in fact be harbingers of future regurgitation. Early in the course of mitral regurgitation from chronic valve disease the murmur may not, in fact, last the entire duration of systole. With progressive deterioration of the mitral valve leaflets or with superimposed rupture of chordae tendineae, the murmur becomes holosystolic. Sudden increases in murmur intensity may be associated with the onset or exacerbation of systemic hypertension or ruptured chordae tendineae. In dogs the loudness of the murmur has been correlated with the severity of the disease and prognosis (i.e., the louder the murmur, the worse the valve disease and the shorter the survival). Chronic valve disease (endocardiosis) is by far the most common cause of regurgitant murmurs (or any murmur) in small or medium-sized dogs greater than 5 years of age and is occasionally seen in old cats (mitral insufficiency in cats is much more likely to be associated with systemic hypertension or hypertrophic cardiomyopathy).

✳ **KEY POINT** The most common murmur in older dogs is caused by mitral valve disease.

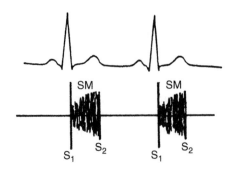

Figure 2-9 Holosystolic murmur (SM) of myxomatous degeneration of the mitral valve with severe mitral valve prolapse.

> ✳ **KEY POINT** A sudden increase in the intensity of the murmur of mitral insufficiency in an older dog should prompt systemic blood pressure measurement, because the murmur intensity often increases dramatically with the onset of hypertension.

Auscultatory clues in severe degenerative mitral valve disease are as follows:

- Loud (grade III or more) holosystolic murmur (Figure 2-9).
- Murmur typically loudest at the left cardiac apex, with wide radiation determined by the direction of blood regurgitation and factors including the coupling of the heart to the chest wall.
- S_3 or S_4 may be present if heart failure is imminent or present.
- Midsystolic click or clicks can be obscured by the loud murmur.

Ruptured Chordae Tendineae. Chordal rupture may occur with chronic degenerative valve disease (endocardiosis), with severe systemic hypertension, or rarely with bacterial endocarditis or blunt chest trauma. Depending on their number and size (primary versus secondary or tertiary chords), ruptured chordae tendineae generally cause the sudden onset or exacerbation of a harsh, loud (grade III or more) holosystolic (or long systolic) murmur, loudest at the left apex, often accompanied by dramatic clinical signs of congestive heart failure that can be refractory to even aggressive therapy. An S_3 (more commonly) or S_4 (if in regular sinus rhythm) may be present. Murmurs in ruptured chordae tendineae are as follows:

- Sudden onset or exacerbation of harsh, loud (grade III or more) holosystolic murmur, frequently enveloping S_1 and S_2 (Figure 2-10).
- Murmur typically loudest at cardiac apex, with radiation pattern variable depending on which chordae rupture.
- S_3 or S_4 (when in regular sinus rhythm) may be present.

Dilated Cardiomyopathy. The systolic regurgitant murmur associated with dilated cardiomyopathy may be caused by dilation of the mitral valve annulus or papillary muscle dysfunction, both of which potentially result in mitral valve incompetence in the face of relatively normal-appearing valve leaflets. Murmurs in this clinical setting are usually early

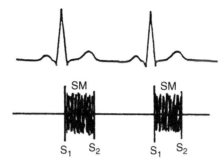

Figure 2-10 Holosystolic murmur (SM) of ruptured chordae tendineae.

systolic, plateau shaped, or occasionally decrescendo, with their PMI at the left apex. The murmur is usually not as loud as in patients with myxomatous degeneration of the mitral valve. Dilated or hypertrophic cardiomyopathy in cats can disrupt the normal mitral valve anatomy, causing a regurgitant murmur as well.

Auscultatory clues to mitral insufficiency secondary to dilated cardiomyopathy are as follows:

- Regurgitant systolic murmur with PMI at L5-6 ICS.
- Murmur usually relatively soft (grade I to III/VI).
- Heart sound intensity often decreased.
- S_3 (more commonly) or S_4 (in sinus rhythm) sometimes present.
- Arrhythmias, especially atrial fibrillation, often present; this results in variation in loudness of heart sounds and the murmur.

> ✳ **KEY POINT** Murmurs caused by right-sided heart disease are often louder on inspiration, whereas murmurs caused by left-sided heart disease are often louder on expiration.

Tricuspid Regurgitation

The systolic murmur of significant tricuspid regurgitation is typically holosystolic and may resemble that of mitral regurgitation in timing and quality. It is heard best over the tricuspid valve area. The loudness and duration of the murmur may vary, depending on the magnitude of regurgitation, but in general the murmur of tricuspid insufficiency is less intense (loud) than comparable amounts of mitral insufficiency (the pressure driving the abnormal blood flow in tricuspid regurgitation is normally less than one third of the driving pressure in mitral regurgitation). Tricuspid insufficiency is most commonly associated with myxomatous degeneration of the tricuspid valve, which complicates approximately 30% of cases of mitral valve endocardiosis or chronic valvular disease in dogs. Severe mitral regurgitation with radiation to the tricuspid valve area can be difficult to differentiate by auscultation alone from combined mitral and tricuspid insufficiency. Other acquired causes of tricuspid insufficiency include pulmonary hypertension secondary to respiratory disease or heartworm disease. The most common congenital causes of tricuspid insufficiency are tricuspid valve dysplasia (mostly in Labrador Retrievers), and as a secondary finding in severe pulmonic stenosis or pulmonary hypertension from any cause.

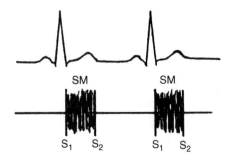

Figure 2-11 Holosystolic murmur (SM) of tricuspid regurgitation.

✳ **KEY POINT** The murmur of tricuspid insufficiency is softer than that of mitral insufficiency with comparable degrees of insufficiency.

Auscultatory clues in tricuspid regurgitation are as follows:

- Holosystolic murmur (Figure 2-11).
- Murmur typically loudest in tricuspid region (right apex).
- S_3 and S_4 usually not present (right-sided S_3 may be present with heart failure).
- The systolic murmur may exhibit respiratory variation in loudness, with accentuation during inspiration.
- Persistent splitting of S_2 may be audible if pulmonary hypertension or heartworm disease is the cause of the valvular insufficiency.

Ventricular Septal Defect

The auscultatory findings in VSD are determined by the size and location of the septal defect and the pulmonary vascular resistance, because these factors primarily determine the amount, direction, and velocity of blood flow from the normally high-pressure left ventricle into the normally low-pressure right ventricle during systole. Because of the large and constant pressure gradient between the ventricles during systole, the murmur of VSD is generally plateau shaped or regurgitant quality. With small to moderate-sized defects and normal to mildly elevated pulmonary vascular resistance (systolic pressure of 50 mm Hg or less in the pulmonary artery), the systolic murmur is typically loud (grade III to V), holosystolic, and medium to high pitched with a harsh quality and a plateau configuration. If pulmonary hypertension accompanies a defect, the murmur may be audible only in early systole. The murmur is usually loudest at the right sternal border, but great individual variation exists in the associated heart sounds and murmur.

Auscultatory clues in moderate-sized congenital VSD with moderate to large left-to-right shunt are as follows:

- Harsh, loud (grade III to V) holosystolic murmur, typically plateau-shaped configuration (Figure 2-12).
- Murmur loudest at the right sternal border.
- S_1 typically normal.
- S_2 may be perceived as normal, or a split may be audible with normal respiratory variation.

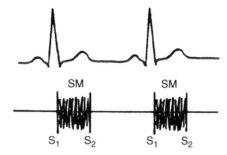

Figure 2-12 **Holosystolic murmur (SM) of congenital ventricular septal defect.**

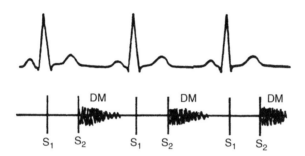

Figure 2-13 **Diastolic murmur (DM) in a dog with vegetative endocarditis of the aortic valve.**

- The middiastolic, low-pitched murmur (caused by high flow across the mitral valve) often heard in humans with VSD is usually not appreciated in dogs or cats.
- Occasionally a soft (grade I to II) systolic ejection murmur may be heard in the pulmonic area, secondary to high flow and relative pulmonic stenosis.

Diastolic Murmurs

Diastolic murmurs are auscultated and recorded between S_2 and S_1 during the phases of ventricular relaxation. A diastolic murmur audible on auscultation almost always indicates significant underlying disease. Diastolic murmurs result from two main mechanisms:

1. Regurgitant flow across incompetent aortic or pulmonic semilunar valves.
2. Forward flow across stenotic mitral or tricuspid AV valves.

Aortic regurgitation is the most commonly recognized diastolic murmur in dogs and cats. Aortic regurgitation causes diastolic murmurs that begin with or immediately after A_2 and are typically high frequency (high pitched), blowing in quality, and decrescendo in configuration (Figure 2-13). These murmurs are best auscultated with the diaphragm of the stethoscope, and soft murmurs of aortic regurgitation are heard best by laying the animal on top of the stethoscope, with the diaphragm up in the left armpit. The most common cause of aortic regurgitation detectable by auscultation in domestic animals is bacterial endocarditis. Severe systemic hypertension (especially when associated with aortic root dilation) may also cause aortic insufficiency in dogs and cats. Color-flow spectral Doppler studies have documented that some aortic regurgitation often accompanies subaortic stenosis, but this small amount of flow rarely produces a murmur that can be heard on auscultation. The murmur of aortic regurgitation is usually heard best in the region of the aortic valve at the left heart base.

> ✳ **KEY POINT** Diastolic murmurs are rare and most commonly associated with bacterial endocarditis of the aortic valve in dogs.

There is a frequent disparity between the intensity or loudness of the aortic regurgitation murmur and the degree of regurgitation apparent on color-flow Doppler. Severe aortic regurgitation may occur with a relatively soft, short murmur, and moderate aortic regurgitation may cause a murmur that is audible only with the animal lying on the stethoscope as described previously. A loud murmur of aortic regurgitation, however, is almost always associated with a hemodynamically important lesion. When valvular aortic stenosis and aortic regurgitation are combined, both the systolic ejection murmur of aortic stenosis and the diastolic murmur of aortic regurgitation are present, forming a to-and-fro murmur, and S_2 is often difficult to hear (Figure 2-14). This situation is distinct from, but can be confused with, a continuous murmur (see the section on Continuous Murmurs). Aortic regurgitation sometimes accompanies VSDs located just beneath the aortic root, and this combination of murmurs (regurgitant systolic and diastolic murmurs), despite being characterized by a distinct pause between the murmur components similar to those in aortic stenosis and regurgitation, can also be confused with a continuous murmur.

Auscultatory clues in mild to moderate aortic regurgitation are as follows:

- High-pitched, blowing decrescendo diastolic murmur starting with or immediately after A_2, usually grades I to III.
- Diastolic murmur typically loudest over the aortic valve region.
- With moderate aortic regurgitation, S_1 diminished.
- S_2 may be narrowly split (with severe aortic regurgitation, paradoxical S_2 splitting may occur). S_2 may be accentuated (with severe aortic regurgitation or associated aortic stenosis with calcified valve, A_2 is diminished and often not heard).
- Aortic ejection sound may be present.
- Left-sided S_3 may be present.

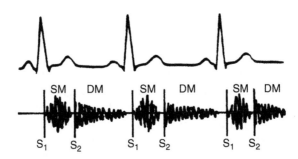

🔊 **Figure 2-14 To-and-fro murmur of aortic stenosis combined with aortic regurgitation.**

The diastolic murmur of *pulmonic regurgitation* usually has pitch and timing similar to the murmur of aortic regurgitation but is far less common. It is usually heard only in the presence of significant pulmonary hypertension, and then it is heard best in the pulmonic valve region (left base), with an accentuated P_2 component of S_2.

Mitral stenosis is a rare congenital defect in dogs, and it is recognized even less frequently in cats. The murmur is characteristically of low frequency, low pitched, and rumbling in quality and is therefore difficult to hear even with the bell of the stethoscope lightly applied to the chest wall with just enough pressure to make a skin seal at the left apex. In contrast with the diastolic murmur of aortic regurgitation, which usually begins immediately after the second heart sound, in mitral stenosis a distinct delay in onset of the murmur follows S_2.

Tricuspid stenosis is another rare congenital defect. The diastolic murmur of tricuspid stenosis is best auscultated over the tricuspid valve area (right apex). The murmur is similar to the mitral stenosis murmur but is typically even softer and of shorter duration. It may be accentuated during inspiration.

Continuous Murmurs

Continuous murmurs are long murmurs that include the entire period of systole and continue beyond the second sound and throughout diastole. Continuous murmurs are usually caused by abnormal blood flow between parts of the arterial and venous circulation that are not normally connected by large vessels (e.g., PDA and other arteriovenous connections). Rarely, continuous murmurs are caused by severe narrowing of the aorta or pulmonary arteries that occur distal to the aortic or pulmonic semilunar valves, such that the vessel proximal to the narrowing (which remains pressurized throughout systole and diastole) is connected to the low-pressure portion of the vessel distal to the narrowing.

Patent ductus arteriosus is a congenital lesion that is the most common cause of a pathologic or organic continuous murmur. It is the most common congenital defect in dogs (although far less common in cats, it is still the most common cause of continuous murmurs in cats). Arbitrarily, the continuous murmur of PDA can be considered to start with S_1 and reach maximal loudness at or slightly before S_2. After S_2 the intensity of the sound diminishes (the decrescendo portion of the murmur) as diastole progresses toward the next S_1. The classic murmur of PDA is loud (up to grade VI), of medium pitch, and heard best at the left side of the base (Figure 2-15). The diastolic component tends to be fairly localized,

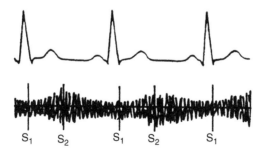

S_1 S_2 S_1 S_2 S_1

Figure 2-15 **Continuous murmur in a Poodle with a patent ductus arteriosus.**

although the systolic component may radiate widely. The overall impression is often similar to putting an ear up to a large conch shell and then moving the shell closer and slightly farther away from the ear; the effect simulates the late systolic peak and diastolic decrescendo portion of the murmur. The diastolic component may sometimes taper off to become inaudible at the very end of diastole, but it never stops abruptly—the auditory impression is one of a distant blowing quality murmur that never abruptly ends in a period of total silence. The murmur is also frequently described as a "machinery" murmur, proceeding continuously from systole into diastole with no periods of silence in between. The loudness and duration of the murmur are directly related to the pressure gradient between the aorta and pulmonary artery. When pulmonary hypertension is present (a rare event in dogs), the intensity of the diastolic component decreases and the intensity of S_2 increases in proportion to the pulmonary pressures. If the direction of the shunt is actually reversed (from right to left, instead of left to right—more commonly the result of retained fetal pulmonary circulation in the dog, as opposed to acquired pulmonary hypertension from enhanced blood flow), the diastolic component disappears and the systolic component at the left side of the base becomes faint or possibly even absent. PDA is most commonly an isolated lesion but may complicate other congenital lesions (e.g., VSD).

> ✳ **KEY POINT** The continuous murmur of a PDA can be quite localized to the heart base, and if you auscultate only over the mitral valve area, you may hear only a systolic murmur of concurrent mitral insufficiency.

Auscultatory clues in PDA are as follows:

- Usually loud, continuous, "machinery" murmur, loudest at the left heart base, often associated with a thrill.
- Systolic component often radiates extensively.
- Systolic regurgitant murmur often heard at the left apex (secondary to mitral regurgitation).
- Long-standing PDA may cause atrial fibrillation, which makes the continuous murmur much more difficult to recognize. Atrial fibrillation occurring in female German Shepherd dogs and Shelties of any age should prompt a thorough search for PDA.

Rare causes of organic or pathologic continuous murmurs include the following:

- Aortic pulmonary window with left-to-right shunt.
- Arteriovenous fistula.
- Sinus of Valsalva or coronary artery aneurysm rupture into the right side of the heart.
- Coarctation of aorta (severe).
- Pulmonary artery branch stenosis.

Summary

Accurate recognition and communication of the timing and other auscultatory characteristics of heart sounds and murmurs is a key step in establishing a working cardiac diagnosis. The characteristics of heart sounds and murmurs are shown in Figure 2-16.

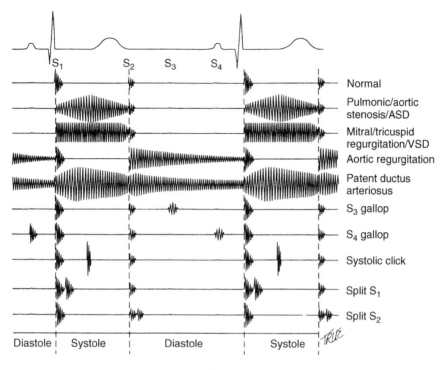

Figure 2-16 Cardiac cycle with electrocardiogram and phonocardiogram schematized. Both normal and abnormal sounds are included. *ASD,* Atrial septal defect; *VSD,* ventricular septal defect. *(From Atkins CE: Abnormal heart sounds. In Allen DG, editor: Small animal medicine, Philadelphia, 1991, Lippincott Williams & Wilkins.)*

● Posttest 2

Part A

1. As the severity of pulmonic stenosis increases from mild to moderate, the murmur intensity _____.
   a. increases
   b. decreases
   c. stays the same
   d. None of the above

2. Subaortic stenosis is a relatively common congenital heart defect in dogs. Which of the following statements is true?
   a. Subaortic stenosis is common in Newfoundland dogs and Golden Retrievers.
   b. The pathologic lesion of subaortic stenosis may worsen though the first year of life.
   c. The murmur intensity may increase through the first year of life.
   d. All of the above statements are true.

3. Which of the following statements is true about the murmur of patent ductus arteriosus?
   a. The murmur is usually heard best on the right hemithorax.
   b. The murmur is usually continuous in the dog.
   c. The murmur gets louder if pulmonary hypertension (high blood pressure in the pulmonary artery) is present.
   d. The murmur gets louder if systemic hypotension (low blood pressure in the aorta) is present.

4. The term "machinery murmur" means that the murmur occurs _____.
   a. in systole
   b. in diastole
   c. continuously
   d. None of the above

5. The murmur of an atrial septal defect is caused by shunting of blood between the left atrium and the right atrium.
   a. True
   b. False

6. Innocent murmurs are _____.
   a. usually soft (grade I-II/VI)
   b. usually heard best at the heart base
   c. usually heard in young animals
   d. All of the above

7. You are listening carefully to a dog in a quiet room, and after listening for a time over the left cardiac apex, you hear a soft systolic murmur. This murmur is heard nowhere else on the chest. What grade is the murmur?
   a. I/VI
   b. II/VI
   c. III/VI
   d. IV/VI

8. A diamond-shaped systolic murmur is heard best at the left heart base. Your differential diagnosis should *not* include which of the following heart defects?
   a. Tricuspid regurgitation
   b. VSD
   c. Aortic valve regurgitation
   d. Pulmonic valve stenosis

9. The murmur of mitral valve regurgitation in cats may be heard best _____.
   a. at the left cardiac apex during systole
   b. at the right heart base during systole
   c. at the left sternal border during systole
   d. Both a and c are correct.

10. A 12-year-old Miniature Poodle has been coming to your practice for 3 years, and last year, you noted a grade II/VI systolic plateau-shaped murmur heard best at the left cardiac apex. A chest radiograph performed last year was within normal limits for heart size, and the dog has remained healthy and on all usual preventative medications throughout the year. This year the owner comes to you with a new complaint of increased drinking and urination, and you note on physical exam that the heart murmur is much louder, grade 4/6, still at the left apex. Your work-up should include which of the following tests?
    a. Urinalysis
    b. Serum chemistry panel
    c. Blood pressure measurement
    d. All of the above

Part B

Directions: Part B consists of five unknowns presented on the accompanying website. After determining the correct answers, fill in the appropriate blanks. Pay close attention to the location and timing of the murmurs. Because you are not examining the patient, the location is provided.

1. Aortic area in a Boxer dog. _____

2. Pulmonic area of a female Sheltie. _____

3. Aortic area in a German Shepherd dog. _____

4. Left apex in a male Poodle. _____

5. Left sternal border in a dyspneic cat. _____

3

Arrhythmias

• Pretest 3

1. Atrial fibrillation is most often characterized by a rapid, irregularly irregular rhythm with variable intensity or loudness of the transient heart sounds. Which statement is correct regarding the common auscultatory findings in atrial fibrillation?
   a. The rhythm sounds chaotic because there are more S_2 than S_1 sounds.
   b. The rhythm sounds chaotic because there are often more S_1 than S_2 sounds.
   c. The rhythm sounds chaotic because there is always an S_3 or S_4 sound present.
   d. The rhythm sounds chaotic because there are perfectly regular pauses between S_2 and the next S_1.

2. Which of the following rhythm pairs can you reasonably expect to be able to differentiate from each other on auscultation?
   a. Paroxysmal atrial tachycardia from paroxysmal ventricular tachycardia.
   b. Low-grade second-degree AV block from sinus arrhythmia.
   c. Atrial fibrillation from sinus arrhythmia.
   d. Sinus rhythm with ventricular premature complexes from sinus rhythm with supraventricular premature complexes.

3. Which statement below best characterizes respiratory sinus arrhythmia?
   a. The heart rate is usually less than 140/minute, and it slows down noticeably when the animal inhales.
   b. The heart rate is usually greater than 160/minute, slowing by more than 10% when the animal inhales.
   c. The heart rate is usually greater than 160/minute, and it slows noticeably on exhalation.
   d. The heart rate is usually less than 140/minute, and it slows noticeably on exhalation.

4. Which of the following statements is true with respect to S_4?
   a. S_4 is often heard in atrial fibrillation because the heart muscle is dilated and relatively stiff (noncompliant) at high heart rates.
   b. S_4 is associated with excess ventricular stiffness but is never heard in atrial fibrillation.
   c. S_4 occurs at the very beginning of diastole and is associated with early ventricular filling.
   d. S_4 is often normal in young cats.

5. Sinus bradycardia is often associated with which of the following physical exam findings or conditions?
   a. Hypothermia
   b. Fever
   c. Hyperthermia
   d. Anxiety

Abbreviations

APC	Atrial premature complex	S_1	First heart sound
AV	Atrioventricular	S_2	Second heart sound
ECG	Electrocardiogram	S_3	Third heart sound
PAT	Paroxysmal atrial tachycardia	S_4	Fourth heart sound
PVT	Paroxysmal ventricular tachycardia	**VPC**	Ventricular premature complex

Auscultation of Selected Arrhythmias

Arrhythmias are most accurately diagnosed by electrocardiography. The first clue that an animal has an arrhythmia, however, is often found on auscultation. Some arrhythmias have distinctive auscultatory findings, whereas others are indistinguishable on auscultation. Any time an unexplained irregularity in heart rate or rhythm is detected on auscultation, an electrocardiogram (ECG) is indicated. The auscultatory findings of a few selected common or clinically important arrhythmias are discussed here.

> ✳ **KEY POINT** Auscultation provides the first clue to the presence of an arrhythmia and in some cases the rhythm diagnosis. When an arrhythmia is auscultated or suspected, however, an ECG should always be obtained to confirm the diagnosis.

Sinus rhythm is a regular rhythm (in which the rate of spontaneous depolarization of the normally functioning sinus node controls the heart rate) characterized by a monotonous S_1-S_2 cadence in which the time between successive S_1s varies by less than 10% with respiration, the relationship between S_1 and S_2 remains constant, and the heart rate stays between relatively well-defined parameters (approximately 60 to 160 beats/minute in dogs, 140 to 210 beats/minute in cats). Sinus rhythm is a normal finding in dogs and cats.

> ✳ **KEY POINT** The most common heart rhythm irregularity heard in dogs is sinus arrhythmia, which is normal.

Sinus arrhythmia, like sinus rhythm, is generated by the spontaneous depolarization of the sinus node, but in sinus arrhythmia the node depolarizes in a regularly irregular pattern (i.e., there is an identifiable pattern to the irregularity) at a normal or slow heart rate. The patterned irregularity is associated with waxing and waning vagal tone, often but not always visibly associated with the phases of respiration. On inspiration vagal tone decreases, which increases the heart rate. The degree of irregularity can be increased by conditions that increase vagal tone. These include respiratory and some gastrointestinal, ocular, or other disturbances that potentially affect vagal tone. Respiratory sinus arrhythmia is normal and common in dogs but uncommon in normal cats, in which this finding is frequently associated with bronchitis or asthma.

> ✳ **KEY POINT** An arrhythmia auscultated in a cat often indicates cardiac disease, because sinus arrhythmia is uncommon in this species.

Auscultatory and physical findings in sinus arrhythmia include the following:

- Normal or slow heart rate.
- Regularly irregular rhythm.
- Heart rate that varies with respiration, increasing on inspiration.
- Sometimes a slight variation in pulse quality; however, no pulse deficits.

Associated clinical conditions are as follows:

- Normal in dogs.
- Accentuated by conditions that increase vagal tone (respiratory and gastrointestinal disorders) in dogs.
- Bronchial asthma in cats.

> ✳ **KEY POINT** Not all regular rhythms are normal (e.g., ventricular tachycardia), and not all irregular rhythms are abnormal (e.g., sinus arrhythmia in dogs).

Atrial fibrillation is generally characterized by a rapid, irregularly irregular rhythm. In atrial fibrillation, depolarization of the sinus node no longer controls the heart rate. Instead, multiple reentrant loops generated in the atria impinge on the atrioventricular (AV) node, which conducts the impulses from the atria at a rate determined by the balance of sympathetic and parasympathetic tone on the AV node. Because of the variable heart rate (and variable ventricular filling and strength of muscle contraction that it causes), the loudness of the heart sounds also varies dramatically from beat to beat. So-called short-cycle (rapid) heartbeats at high overall heart rates in atrial fibrillation often cause pulse deficits (S_1 occurring without a subsequent S_2, because the weak ventricular contraction generated on the short-cycle beat is strong enough to raise the pressure in the ventricle sufficiently to close the mitral and tricuspid valve but is too weak to overcome the resistance to ejection of blood into the aorta and pulmonary artery, so that S_2 never occurs on that beat). Audio examples of atrial fibrillation in both a dog and a cat are provided.

Typical auscultatory and physical findings in atrial fibrillation (Figure 3-1) include the following:

- Rapid heart rate.
- Irregularly irregular rhythm.
- Irregularity not associated with respiration.
- Variably loud heart sounds.
- Combination of irregular rhythm and variably loud heart sounds that produces an auscultatory experience analogous to listening to tennis shoes being tumble dried.
- Pulse quality usually decreased, irregular in fullness, and with frequent pulse deficits at high rates.
- Heartbeats that are difficult to correlate with arterial pulses.

Associated clinical conditions are as follows:

- Dilated cardiomyopathy in dogs.
- Hypertrophic or restrictive cardiomyopathy in cats.
- Severe mitral regurgitation secondary to valvular disease in dogs.

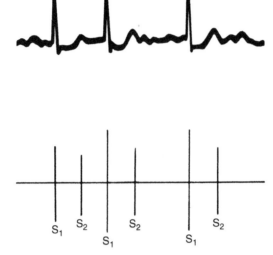

Figure 3-1 Atrial fibrillation in a Doberman Pinscher. Note the irregularity in the rhythm and the variability in the intensity of the heart sounds.

 KEY POINT Atrial fibrillation results in a rapid, irregularly irregular rhythm with varying loudness of heart sounds and pulse deficits.

Auscultatory findings with high-grade second-degree or complete heart block generally include a slow heart rate. S_1 and S_2 may occur at regular intervals at a slow rate, or periods of longer pauses may take place, depending on the ventricular escape rate and AV nodal conduction. The loudness of the first and second heart sounds may vary somewhat owing to variable ventricular filling. S_4 may be audible in association with atrial contraction, and the rate of S_4 may be much faster than the S_1-S_2 cadence, which can be confusing. The S_4-S_4 interval may be regular or irregular depending on whether the underlying rhythm is a sinus rhythm or sinus arrhythmia. There is no association between the S_1-S_2 cadence and S_4.

Auscultatory and physical findings in complete heart block (Figure 3-2) include the following:

- Rhythm that may be slow and regular if S_4 is not audible or may seem irregular and chaotic if S_4 is audible.
- Pulses regular even if the rhythm sounds chaotic. Arterial pulses coincide with S_1. S_4, if part of the audible rhythm, does not produce a femoral pulse.
- Large jugular pulsations often visible at irregular intervals when atrial contraction serendipitously occurs during ventricular systole (called a cannon A wave—remember that in complete heart block the ventricles are being depolarized independent of the atria, so there is no guarantee that atrial contraction will precede ventricular contraction).

Associated clinical conditions are as follows:

- Idiopathic AV nodal fibrosis or degeneration in geriatric animals.
- Cardiomyopathy in cats.

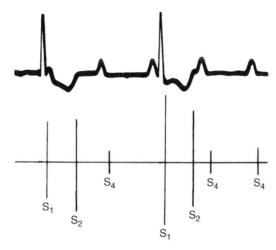

Figure 3-2 Complete atrioventricular block in a 12-year-old Cocker Spaniel. When a P wave occurs before the QRS complex (second complex), the first heart sound is accentuated. Note that an S_4 may be associated with the nonconducted P waves.

- Neoplastic infiltration into the AV node.
- Endocarditis or myocarditis.

✳ **KEY POINT** An S_4 dissociated from the S_1-S_2 cadence suggests AV block.

 Ventricular premature complexes (VPCs) should always be suspected when a heartbeat occurs prematurely (i.e., the heart rhythm is audibly interrupted by a premature beat and subsequent slight pause in the rhythm).

Auscultatory and physical findings with VPCs (Figure 3-3) include the following:

- A regular or regularly irregular rhythm that is interrupted by a premature beat.
- A premature beat that is difficult to hear or inaudible, so that the pause following the premature beat can easily be misinterpreted as a "dropped beat."
- A premature beat that fails to produce a palpable femoral pulse (pulse deficit) or produces one of reduced magnitude. The more premature the beat, the weaker the pulse that can be expected. A late diastolic VPC may not produce a perceptible change in pulse quality. Pulse deficits associated with premature ventricular contractions occur more commonly at high heart rates.
- Splitting of heart sounds (S_1 and S_2) may occur owing to asynchronous depolarization and subsequent contraction of the ventricles by the VPC.

Common associated clinical conditions are as follows:

- Cardiomyopathy in dogs and cats.
- Hyperthyroidism in cats.
- Splenic disease (including hemangiosarcoma) in dogs.
- Chest trauma in dogs and rarely in cats.
- Systemic diseases (e.g., gastric torsion, pancreatitis) in dogs.

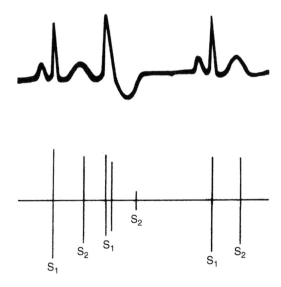

Figure 3-3 Ventricular premature complex (second complex) in a dog. Note the split first heart sound and softer S_2.

VPCs and atrial premature complexes (APCs) cannot reliably be differentiated on the basis of auscultation. Both occur prematurely and can cause pulse deficits. APCs maintain atrial and ventricular synchrony and therefore usually generate a stronger pulse for any given degree of prematurity. This fact, however, is rarely useful in distinguishing the arrhythmias. VPCs may produce a jugular pulse, whereas APCs generally do not, and VPCs are often associated with audible splitting of the first and second heart sound, but this is a subtle finding that may be difficult to appreciate in clinical circumstances.

✳ **KEY POINT** Ventricular premature complexes and atrial premature complexes cannot reliably be differentiated on the basis of auscultation.

Paroxysmal ventricular tachycardia and paroxysmal atrial tachycardia (PVT, PAT) are characterized by bursts of more than three consecutive beats of tachycardia that begin and end abruptly (in contrast, sinus tachycardia classically has a recognizable "warm up" and "cool down" period). Patients may have periods of sinus tachycardia that accelerate quite quickly, however, and can be confused with PAT or PVT on auscultation. PAT and PVT cannot accurately be differentiated by auscultation and require ECG confirmation. In general, tachycardia is termed paroxysmal or nonsustained if it lasts for less than 30 seconds before termination in sinus rhythm.

Auscultatory and physical findings in PAT and PVT (Figure 3-4) include the following:

- Bursts of tachycardia (heart rate up to 400 beats/minute) that begin and end abruptly.
- Isolated premature beats (APC or VPC) may occur during nontachycardic periods.
- Pulses that become weak or absent during tachycardic episodes.

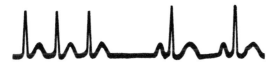

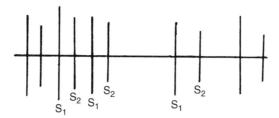

Figure 3-4 Paroxysmal atrial tachycardia (first three complexes) in a 10-year-old Poodle.

Common conditions associated with PAT are as follows:

- Atrial distension secondary to AV valve disease or cardiomyopathy.
- Ventricular preexcitation.
- Systemic, primary noncardiac disease (e.g., renal failure, pancreatitis, snakebite).

Sustained tachycardias are generally defined as those lasting greater than 30 seconds in duration. Sinus tachycardia, ventricular tachycardia, and atrial tachycardia cannot be reliably differentiated based on auscultation. Vagal maneuvers (e.g., ocular or carotid sinus pressure) can help differentiate sinus tachycardia from atrial tachycardia. If the tachycardia breaks abruptly with the vagal maneuver, this supports atrial tachycardia. If the rate gradually slows with the vagal maneuver and then gradually speeds up after the vagal maneuver, this supports sinus tachycardia. Often the vagal maneuver elicits no response, in which case either rhythm is still possible. An ECG should be obtained for any patient with sustained tachycardia.

✳ **KEY POINT** Rapid heart rates are common in cats and are often a normal variant, but diseases such as hyperthyroidism and cardiomyopathy should be considered.

The term "gallop rhythm" is a misnomer; gallop sounds are not necessarily a sign of rhythm disturbance but indicate the presence of extra heart sounds (S_3 and S_4). These extra sounds are sometimes mistaken for an arrhythmia. They are caused by changes in the mechanical function of the heart, rather than the heart's rate or pattern of electrical depolarization, and the ECG rhythm is unaffected.

✳ **KEY POINT** Gallop "rhythms" are extra heart sounds and are not indicative of an arrhythmia.

Posttest 3

Part A

1. Auscultation is often useful in establishing the heart rhythm and identifying rhythm abnormalities. Choose the correct statement.
   a. A rapid, irregular rhythm on auscultation in a large-breed dog is always atrial fibrillation.
   b. An ECG is usually needed to establish a definitive rhythm diagnosis.
   c. Pulse deficits are common in sinus arrhythmia.
   d. Pulse deficits are common in sinus tachycardia.

2. Choose the correct statement regarding premature contractions.
   a. At high heart rates, a premature beat can sometimes cause a nearly inaudible S_1 without a subsequent S_2, resulting in a pause in the rhythm often recognized as a "dropped beat."
   b. At heart rates above 160/minute, it's relatively easy to confuse atrial fibrillation with sinus arrhythmia.
   c. Sinus rhythm interrupted by combinations of paroxysmal ventricular premature beats, ventricular couplets, and isolated VPCs can easily be distinguished from atrial fibrillation.
   d. Atrial premature beats rarely occur in dogs with a heart murmur caused by mitral valve regurgitation.

3. Sinus tachycardia is commonly associated with which of the following conditions?
   a. Fever
   b. Hypothermia
   c. Hypothyroidism
   d. Bronchitis

4. Which of the following diseases is commonly associated with premature ventricular contractions heard on auscultation and confirmed by ECG?
   a. Dilated cardiomyopathy in Doberman Pinschers
   b. Arrhythmogenic right ventricular cardiomyopathy in Boxers
   c. Splenic hemangiosarcoma
   d. All of the above

5. Gallop sounds (S_3, S_4, or a summation gallop) can be difficult to distinguish from which of the following conditions?
   a. Atrial fibrillation
   b. Ventricular premature beat
   c. Midsystolic click
   d. Atrial premature beat

Part B

Directions: Part B consists of four unknowns presented on the accompanying website. After determining the correct answers, fill in the appropriate blanks. Some cases have more than one possible answer.

1. Irish Wolfhound with dilated cardiomyopathy. _____

2. This arrhythmia is heard in a coughing dog with bronchitis. _____

3. This arrhythmia is heard in a German Shepherd that had been hit by a car. _____

4. This arrhythmia is heard in a 5-year-old Doberman Pinscher seen for routine vaccination. _____

4

Lung Sounds

Objectives

Upon completion of this chapter, you should be able to:

1. Understand the origin of normal lung sounds.
2. Appropriately use standard nomenclature for describing respiratory sounds.
3. Understand how lung sounds are transmitted to the chest wall and stethoscope.
4. Recognize the effect of airway, lung, and pleural space disease on lung sounds and breathing patterns.
5. Recognize limitations of lung sounds in diagnosing disease conditions.

• Pretest 4

1. Normal lung sounds originate in _____.
   a. bronchi and alveoli (vesicles)
   b. the entire conducting airway system
   c. the trachea and first few generations of bronchi
   d. small airways that are oriented toward the stethoscope

2. Lung sounds are formed by _____.
   a. turbulent air flow in large bronchi
   b. turbulent air flow in small bronchi
   c. laminar air flow in large bronchi
   d. laminar air flow in small bronchi

3. The accepted term used to indicate an abnormal sound heard in dogs with pulmonary edema is _____.
   a. rales
   b. fine crackles
   c. wet lung sounds
   d. harsh lung sounds

4. The abnormal sound heard in dogs with pulmonary edema described in question 3 is caused by _____.
   a. air bubbling through fluid in alveoli and small airways
   b. air bubbling through fluid in lobar and subsegmental bronchi
   c. abrupt opening of small airways
   d. snapping shut of small airways

5. Compared with rhonchi, wheezes are _____.
   a. higher pitch, audible at the mouth
   b. lower pitch, audible at the mouth
   c. lower pitch, audible only near the source
   d. higher pitch, audible only near the source

Writing in the *Lancet* in 1967, British pulmonologist Paul Forgacs summarized the potential range of sounds made by the lung when he stated that "the sound repertoire of a wet sponge such as the lung is limited." Lung sounds refer to both normal and abnormal sounds that are produced in the larynx, trachea, bronchi, and small airways and auscultated over the thoracic wall. Although everyone agrees that lung sounds are difficult to hear and categorize, there has been little agreement or uniformity in the terminology used to describe the sounds. Part of the difficulty in listening to lung sounds stems from the fact that they are normally soft, low-frequency sounds that are difficult to hear, and part of the difficulty comes from the relative infrequency of the event (breathing) that makes the sounds. Normal respiratory rates in dogs and cats vary between about 10 and 30 breaths/min; if listening to 2 or 3 breaths over the trachea and each of 4 separate locations on each side of the thorax can be considered to constitute the auscultatory part of a complete respiratory examination, it often takes nearly 2 minutes just to listen to the lung sounds of a normal animal. This is a significant amount of time in a busy practice environment, and the temptation to skip a time-consuming, difficult procedure is great. However, without a large mental library of normal lung sounds acquired by carefully listening to hundreds of normal animals, critical evaluation of lung sounds in sick animals becomes nearly impossible. Understanding the basics of how lung sounds are produced and transmitted to the stethoscope is the first step in being able to critically evaluate these sometimes frustrating sounds.

The lung sounds heard by using a stethoscope at the chest wall are affected by a variety of factors, including the characteristics and intensity of the sounds produced in the respiratory tract and the transmission of those sounds to and through the chest wall and the stethoscope itself. Airway structure plays an important role in respiratory sound production, and patterns of airway branching in the thorax have been carefully studied in a number of species. There are also significant effects produced by different breathing patterns (including the amounts of air typically inspired at the beginning versus the end of inspiration or exhaled during the phases of expiration) and breathing frequencies between species that affect the production and transmission of both normal and abnormal lung sounds. In contrast to cardiac auscultation, lung auscultation should always be done using the stethoscope diaphragm, because the diaphragm significantly outperforms the bell at frequencies between 400 and 2000 Hz, the range of interest for most abnormal lung sounds.

Normal Respiratory Sounds

Types of respiratory sounds include *breath*, *tracheal*, and *lung* sounds. Breath sounds are heard at the mouth with or without a stethoscope; tracheal sounds are heard by placing the stethoscope directly over the trachea; and lung sounds are heard with the stethoscope on the chest wall. Normal lung sounds are created by movement of air in the tracheobronchial tree. In general, normal lung sounds are made by turbulent air flow in large (>2 mm diameter) airways. As air moves through the larynx, into the trachea, and down the bronchial tree toward the alveoli, the velocity of the air movement progressively slows (as the total cross-sectional area of the airways increases), and air flow becomes laminar and therefore sound generation is greatly reduced by the third division of bronchi. Although large tubes conduct high-pitched sound well, tubes less than 2 mm in diameter do not—so it is the lung parenchyma that actually conducts the sounds made in the large airways to the pleural surface of the lung.

The lung parenchyma is made up of alveoli, small airways, capillaries, and supporting tissues. Sound generated in the large airways is attenuated in the thorax by three general mechanisms: spreading, absorption by lung and chest wall volume effects, and the reflection of sound waves at the skin surface. Spreading of sound with increasing distance from its source obeys the inverse square law (intensity is inversely proportional to distance squared). Because most lung sound is generated at a central location within or near the mediastinum, lung sound intensity falls as one auscultates farther from the trachea and hilar region. Volume effects cause loss of sound wave energy to friction, thermal conduction, and molecular relaxation, effects that also attenuate the sound in proportion to the distance from its source. Lung alveoli act as elastic bubbles, and the loss of sound energy to dynamic deformation of the alveoli is greatest at higher frequencies (pitch) as sound wavelength becomes shorter. Frictional and thermal conduction forces account for a large share of sound attenuation, particularly as frequency (pitch) increases, and the result is that normal lungs act as low-pass filters that are much more efficient at transmitting the low frequencies (<400 Hz) that characterize normal heart and lung sound.

The flesh of the chest wall, particularly adipose tissue, strongly attenuates sound at lower frequencies. As a result, heart sounds and low-frequency lung sounds are much quieter at the chest wall of obese patients. The greatest attenuation of sound occurs secondary to reflection at the skin-atmosphere interface, where less than 1% to 5% (varying with frequency) of sound energy escapes. Because the chest wall has such a profound effect on the transmission of lung sounds, clinicians need to consider the animal's body conformation and chest wall thickness (and hair coat) when judging the intensity of lung sounds heard over a patient's chest. For example, it may be almost impossible to hear any lung sounds in some obese cats, especially in the absence of cardiopulmonary disease. Veterinary clinicians must construct a mental library of normal respiratory sound intensity for all of the species with which they work, as well as for the range of body shapes, sizes, and condition scores found within each of the species.

In sum, only a small fraction of sound generated in the large airways is transmitted to the skin surface because of the effects of spreading, absorption, scattering, and reflection. Transmission to the surface of the chest is highly heterogeneous because of the heterogeneity of the thoracic structures, and in general attenuation becomes more severe as the frequency (pitch) increases. Consequently, higher frequency sounds are regionally restricted, underscoring the importance of choosing an optimal location to hear heart and lung sounds in health and disease.

Based on the modern understanding of the genesis of lung sounds, the vocabulary used to describe them is simple: they may be normal, increased, or decreased. The terms "bronchovesicular" and "vesicular breath sounds" are known now to be mistakes, although the words are still in common use. "Vesicular" implies that sound is made in the alveoli (the vesicles of the lung), which is not true—these sounds are simply large airway sounds that are transmitted through the lung parenchyma and chest wall. In the dog, inspiratory lung sounds generally come from lobar and large subsegmental bronchi, and sounds heard during exhalation are formed in the trachea and the first one to two divisions of bronchi.

Just before lung auscultation it is useful to first observe the animal's conformation, body condition score, and respiratory pattern, then listen (without the stethoscope) for any abnormal noise audible at the mouth, and finally auscultate directly over the trachea. Because there is no lung tissue between the stethoscope and trachea and there is comparatively very little variation in the thickness of neck tissue between individuals within a species, the sound heard there is a useful reference point to serve as a basis for comparison and interpretation of lung sounds. Because there is no lung tissue attenuation of sound, the tracheal sounds are louder and higher-pitched, containing more energy in frequencies between 1000 and 3000 Hz than the normal lung, which is mostly <400 Hz and almost entirely <1000 Hz auscultated at the chest wall. The intensity of normal lung sounds is best judged by carefully listening to a few breaths in comparable locations on each side of the chest of a standing animal and comparing the intensity and timing of the sounds heard in comparable locations on the left and right hemithorax. Allowances must be made for the animal's body conformation and condition, as well as for any asymmetries in the hair coat, chest wall structure, or posture. The respiratory pattern has a large effect: high air velocity (as seen with panting or increased respiratory effort) produces greater turbulent flow in smaller airways than normal tidal breathing, resulting in louder and "harsher" (higher pitch) sounds that are characterized simply as "increased."

Normal lung sounds differ in pitch (frequency), loudness (intensity), and timing when heard over various parts of the animal's chest. No matter where the sounds are made (larynx, trachea, or central bronchi), turbulent air flow causes the airway walls to vibrate, and those vibrations create sound that travels through large airways into the adjacent tissue. Conditions that increase the velocity of air flow (narrowed airways, increased air flow rate) increase the amount of turbulence and the intensity or loudness of sounds produced. Conversely, clinical situations that reduce the velocity of air flow tend to reduce the amount of turbulence and the amount of sound produced. Airway anatomy plays a significant role; for example, the loudest lung region in a normal dog is over the right middle lung lobe because of the conformation and orientation of its lobar bronchus.

Disease states alter the sound transmission characteristics of the thorax and yield distinct changes. In general, when disease states replace normal alveoli with consolidation, infiltration, or fibrosis the lung becomes a more efficient transmitter of high-frequency sound and lung sounds are increased. As lung water or tissue content increases with edema, inflammation, or infiltration, attenuation by lung volume effects is diminished and the sounds heard at the surface are increased in both amplitude (they are louder) and pitch (because more high-frequency sound is transmitted to the surface), and these changes can be detected by electronic analysis at very early stages of disease progression, typically long before the development of adventitial sounds. How well a clinician performs at detecting this change is dependent on many factors, including the size of that "mental library" mentioned earlier!

The most extreme example of increased lung sounds is termed "bronchial breathing," when the sound heard over a given region is similar to that heard over the trachea. This condition occurs when the lung is completely consolidated. That lung sounds are loudest over a region with no ventilation seems counterintuitive because one is auscultating over a solid, airless area of lung, but in this case the sound created in large bronchi serving ventilated regions of lung is being transmitted more efficiently through that solid consolidated region. This phenomenon is expected whenever there is radiographic evidence of a severe alveolar pattern surrounding a lobar air bronchogram. If the bronchus becomes obliterated by compression or filling with fluid, the lobe loses its acoustical airway connection with the source of sound and lung sounds over the lobe are severely reduced.

Lung sounds may be reduced by slowing air velocity during inspiration and exhalation, as seen in quietly resting animals, many normal cats, or dogs with neuromuscular disorders causing weakness of respiratory muscles. Lung sounds are also reduced by the introduction of air or fluid (e.g., effusion, hemorrhage, pneumothorax) into the pleural space that adds an additional acoustical reflection point between the lung and the stethoscope. In this case, additional sound is lost by increased reflection of sound at the lung–pleural space interface. The intensity of lung sounds heard at the chest wall is usually diminished in animals with clinically significant pleural disease in the regions of the thorax in which the additional acoustical interface is present, for example the dorsal lung fields in a standing dog with pneumothorax or the ventral thorax of a cat with pleural effusion resting in sternal recumbency. Furthermore, the tidal volume in animals with significant pleural disease falls as the pleural disease progresses (despite increasing respiratory effort), decreasing the intensity of the normal lung sounds produced and contributing to the observation that normal lung sounds are difficult to hear in animals with pleural disease.

Abnormal (Adventitial) Lung Sounds

Before Forgacs' ground-breaking research and publications describing the functional basis and clinical correlations of both normal and abnormal lung sounds, physicians and veterinarians used a variety of terms to describe what were thought to be distinctly recognizable kinds of abnormal lung sounds. Kotlikoff and Gillespie writing in 1983 found at least 23 such terms used to modify the basic terms then used for abnormal lung sounds. This finding was reproduced in veterinary medicine by Roudebush in a 1989 survey of 310 veterinary case reports or clinical reviews that found 7 different terms used to qualify breath sounds, 12 to qualify crackles (which were often referred to as "rales"), 7 additional terms to describe other discontinuous sounds (e.g., "moist," "congestion," "fluid sounds," "gurgling," "crepitation," "rattling," "clicks"), and 7 more to describe continuous lung sounds. Those terms are now acknowledged to lack clinical utility, because the sounds they were thought to describe turned out not to be truly recognizable as distinct from one another (this was part of Forgacs' contribution). Continued clinical use of such terms as "wet rales" (or moist, dry, or humid ones) serves now mostly to label practitioners as "hopeless geezers," "clueless clinicians," or both.

At the tenth meeting of the International Lung Sounds Association in 1985 a nomenclature committee agreed that all adventitial (abnormal) lung sounds could and should be described by a scheme that included only the terms crackles (fine and coarse), wheezes, and rhonchi. Each of these terms refers to a group of abnormal lung sounds that can be identified and described acoustically, but none is associated with an absolutely consistent mechanism or location of sound production (Tables 4-1 and 4-2). These terms are fairly widely accepted in veterinary medicine, although some clinicians still use archaic terms like "rales" (generally meaning fine crackles) and "harsh" (meaning increased) lung sounds. Adventitial lung sounds are abnormal lung sounds that are superimposed on normal (or increased/decreased) lung sounds. The three distinct kinds of adventitial sounds recognized by the International Lung Sounds Association are also recognized in dogs and cats.

▶ Fine Crackles

Fine crackles are short-duration (<20 msec), high-pitched (>800 Hz), rapidly damped, nonmusical lung sounds. Although this sound was historically attributed to the presence of "fluid in the alveoli or airways," it is now known that the phenomenon usually has nothing to do with edema fluid within the pulmonary air space. Fine crackles are caused by the same processes that cause increased lung sounds and represent the explosive opening of small airways creating a brief high-pitched noise. Small airways (without a complete cartilage ring) may collapse secondary to increased lung water or cellular

■ **Table 4-1** Summary of the Genesis and Acoustic Characteristics and Timing of Normal and Abnormal Lung Sounds

Lung Sound	Acoustic Characteristics	Timing
Normal lung sounds	Low frequency, quiet Loudest at the right middle lung lobe in normal dogs	Louder on inspiration
Tracheal sounds	Higher frequency, louder	Both inspiration and expiration
Increased lung sounds	Louder and includes higher frequencies (higher pitch)	May be louder during both inspiration and exhalation
Decreased lung sounds	Quieter, and includes lower frequencies (softer pitch)	May be impossible to hear, particularly on exhalation
Adventitial Lung Sounds		
Coarse crackles	<50 msec, 7-800 Hz, heard at mouth and trachea as well as thorax	Inspiration, expiration, or both
Fine crackles	<20 msec, >800 Hz, heard over thorax and sometimes at trachea, but not at the mouth	Early or late inspiration
Wheezes	Longer duration (>80 msec), high pitch (>1000 Hz), soft or loud	Usually on exhalation but may occur during inspiration or both
Rhonchi	Longer duration (>100 msec), low pitch (<2-300 Hz), loud	Inspiration, expiration, or both

■ **Table 4-2** Summary of Expected Lung Sound Findings in a Variety of Common Cardiopulmonary Conditions of Dogs and Cats

Condition	Amplitude Compared with Normal Lung Sounds*	Adventitial Sounds
Pulmonary edema	Usually louder (unless the animal takes shallow breaths because of fatigue)	Usually present (end-inspiratory fine crackles, with or without wheezes)
Pleural effusion	Quieter	Usually absent, depending on cause (e.g., can coexist with pulmonary edema)
Pneumothorax	Quieter	Usually absent
Bronchitis	Normal to increased	Usually absent, can be present (inspiratory or inspiratory and expiratory coarse crackles or wheezes)
Pneumonia	Increased unless there is obliteration of lobar bronchus	Usually present (coarse crackles, with or without wheezes or rhonchi)

*Assuming that the patient is not fatigued to the point that the tidal volume is diminished.

infiltration that counters the traction and scaffolding effects of the alveolar septae, which normally maintain the patency of small conducting airways through exhalation. Small airways may also be obstructed secondary to the presence of airway exudate that obliterates the lumen without producing actual collapse of the airway wall. The popping open of small airways that causes fine crackles to form in the lung may occur during any portion of inspiration, depending on the underlying pathologic cause of the pressure changes required to produce sudden airway opening or compression. When hundreds of small airways pop open nearly simultaneously, the result is a sound that is similar to that heard when pulling Velcro® apart. Another fair approximation of crackles can be produced by finely rubbing a small lock of hair back and forth between the thumb and index finger, as close to the ear canal as possible.

Fine crackles occur most often at the beginning or end of inspiration. Although they generally indicate the presence of a pulmonary pathology in small animals, the sound itself has no pathognomonic clinical correlates: animals with bronchitis, pulmonary edema, pneumonia, or pulmonary fibrosis may all have crackles (although the timing and intensity of their crackles may differ, and their clinical presentations may be quite distinct). Early inspiratory crackles are often associated with obstructive lung diseases such as chronic bronchitis and asthma. Mid- to late-inspiratory crackles may be associated with restrictive pulmonary disease such as interstitial fibrosis, pneumonia, and pulmonary edema. Animals with shallow breathing owing to restrictive lung disease or respiratory fatigue may not be able to increase their lung volume enough to open these airways, explaining the absence of fine crackles sometimes observed in animals with radiographic evidence of severe infiltrate or edema. One trick to increase the ability to identify crackles in these animals (if their condition permits) is to induce cough by tracheal palpation. If they are strong enough to cough, the inspiration immediately preceding the cough will be relatively deep, often increasing the lung volume sufficiently to produce fine crackles. The deeper breath usually reveals increased lung sounds as well. The cough itself will sometimes reveal rhonchi (see below) associated with intrathoracic collapse of large airways and/or mobilization of exudate in the trachea and large bronchi.

✳ **KEY POINT** Presence of fine crackles does not confirm the presence of heart failure, because fine crackles are heard with both primary lung disease and heart failure.

▶ Coarse Crackles

Coarse crackles are usually lower-pitched (≈700-800 Hz) and longer in duration (<50 msec) than fine crackles, and represent rupture of fluid membranes in the mouth, pharynx, larynx, trachea, and first few generations of bronchi. Although these are heard well over the thorax, they are differentiated from fine crackles by the fact one can easily hear them over the trachea and at the mouth (with or without a stethoscope). When a person or animal "sounds congested" as you approach, you are hearing coarse crackles. Coarse crackles are found in animals with tracheobronchitis or other inflammatory disorders of the large airways.

✳ **KEY POINT** Coarse crackles indicate the presence of fluid in large airways; this may be caused by severe heart failure but also by tracheobronchitis and other disorders.

▶ Wheezes

Compared with crackles, wheezes are much longer duration (>80-100 msec), relatively high-pitched (often >1000 Hz), sinusoidal (musical) sounds associated with narrowing of an airway and are caused either by vibrations of small bronchial walls or by vibrations set up between a structure (e.g., a mucus plug or a mass) and a bronchial wall. Although small airway constriction associated with asthma provides the classic clinical cause of wheezing, wheezes can accompany other conditions that cause either temporary or permanent small airway narrowing (including but not limited to pulmonary edema, pneumonia, bronchitis, fibrosis, or intraluminal or compressive neoplasia). The presence of wheezes should be taken as a sign of a pulmonary pathology with involvement of bronchi, but they are not pathognomonic for any single disease and they are not all caused by a uniform pathophysiologic mechanism.

> ✳ **KEY POINT** Wheezes should be taken as a sign of small airway disease, but they are not pathognomonic for any single disease.

Rhonchi

Rhonchi (the singular form of the word is rhonchus) are also long-duration sounds (>100 msec), but in contrast to wheezes they are low pitched (<2-300 Hz) because they are caused by either vibration of large airways (similar to a wheeze, but in the pharynx, larynx, or trachea) or by the rupture of air-fluid interfaces (e.g., breathing through significant amounts of exudate in a large airway). Rhonchi are often snoring-type sounds that are easily heard at both the trachea and over the thoracic wall. Their presence indicates either:

▶ • Upper airway collapse.
▶ • The presence of abnormal accumulations of secretions in large airways.

Stridor is the term used to describe a harsh sound generally heard at a distance during inspiration (or sometimes exhalation) and caused by laryngeal or other large airway obstruction that results in near-occlusion. Expiratory stridor can sometimes be heard with ▶ intrathoracic tracheal collapse. Situations that increase respiratory rate and depth (e.g., exercise, excitement) may bring on clinically obvious stridor in an animal with normal respiratory sounds at rest. Stertor is the term generally used to describe the low-pitched inspiratory sounds associated with nasopharyngeal obstruction owing to elongated soft palate, redundant pharyngeal tissue, or weak pharyngeal musculature. Brachycephalic airway syndrome is the most common cause of inspiratory stridor and stertor in dogs. Laryngeal paralysis is a common cause of inspiratory stertor during normal respiratory effort in several breeds, including Labrador Retrievers, Bouvier des Flandres, Siberian ▶ Huskies, Dalmatians, Rottweilers, St. Bernards, and Newfoundlands. When presented during an obstructive crisis the stertor is usually replaced by stridor, a much higher pitched inspiratory noise created by vigorous inspiratory effort against a tightly closed (by ▶ the marked inspiratory effort) laryngeal orifice. Laryngeal paralysis generally affects middle-aged to older animals, sometimes in association with hypothyroidism. Some patients with laryngeal paralysis also have a history of a change in bark quality.

※ **KEY POINT** Stridor usually indicates the presence of a marked narrowing of an airway structure, as seen in laryngeal paralysis or tracheal collapse. Stertor is a lower frequency sound heard with less severe obstruction and is caused by vibration of large structures such as the soft palate or pharyngeal wall.

Percussion

Percussion is used to elicit areas of dullness (hyporesonance, caused for example by areas of lung consolidation or pleural effusion) or hyperresonance (as might occur with pneumothorax or feline asthma). Percussion has an undeserved reputation as an impractical or inaccurate diagnostic test. The sound produced when a body surface is struck is termed a "percussion note." These notes vary, producing a scale of resonance that ranges from flat notes (relatively high-frequency notes of short duration and little or no resonance) to tympanic notes (low-frequency notes of long duration and exceptional resonance). Some examples of the underlying tissues that produce the most easily discernible of these notes follow, arranged from the most to the least resonant:

- Tympanic—the sound produced by percussion of an air-filled hollow structure.
- Hyperresonant—the sound produced by percussion of pneumothorax or hyperinflated lungs (e.g., feline asthma).
- Resonant—the sound produced by percussion over normal lungs.
- Hyporesonant—the sound produced by percussion over lungs with increased fluid density (e.g., pulmonary edema).
- Dull—the sound produced by percussion over a significant pleural effusion.
- Flat—the sound produced by percussion of the gluteal muscles.

■ **Table 4-3** Pathophysiologic Influences on the Transmission and Intensity of Lung Sounds

Pathophysiology	Intensity of Lung Sounds
Deep breathing or high air velocity (panting)	Increased
Shallow breathing	Decreased
Weight gain, thick hair coat, mesomorphic or endomorphic or heavily muscled chest wall, barrel-chested conformation	Decreased
Weight loss, thin hair coat, ectomorphic/deep-chested conformation	Increased
Decreased density of pulmonary parenchyma, usually caused by air trapping, increased functional residual capacity (e.g., asthma, emphysema)	Decreased
Increased density of pulmonary parenchyma caused by interstitial or alveolar infiltrate with cells or fluid (e.g., overhydration, edema, pneumonia, bronchitis)	Increased
Additional sound-reflective interface in the pleural space between the lung and chest wall (e.g., pleural effusion, hemothorax, pneumothorax)	Decreased

With practice on normal animals of varying hair coats, breeds, body conditions, and conformations, the clinician will build a mental library of normal, expected percussion notes and will find it easy to recognize inappropriately hyperresonant or hyporesonant notes associated with pulmonary or pleural pathology. By combining the information available from auscultation of the heart and lungs (intensity of normal lung sounds [Table 4-3] and presence or absence of adventitial lung sounds) with percussion of the thorax, the clinician will dramatically increase his or her diagnostic acumen in emergency situations involving dyspneic animals when radiographs may be contraindicated (Table 4-4).

■ **Table 4-4** Characteristic Physical Examination Findings in Animals with Thoracic Disease

	Lung Sound Intensity	Adventitial Sounds	Percussion Note
Normal lung	Normal	None	Resonant
Pulmonary edema	Increased	Crackles, possible wheezes	Hyporesonant
Asthma	Often decreased	Wheezes	Hyperresonant
Pleural effusion	Softer or absent ventrally, may be increased dorsally*	None	Dull
Pneumothorax	Softer or absent dorsally, may be increased ventrally*	None	Tympanic

*Assuming the animal is standing or in sternal recumbency.

● Posttest 4

Part A

1. Coarse crackles are caused by_____.
   a. opening of small airways
   b. subcutaneous emphysema
   c. mobilization of fluid in large airways
   d. vibration of the walls of large airways

2. The frequency range for normal and most abnormal lung sounds is _____ Hz, respectively.
   a. 400-1000 and less than 400
   b. less than 400 and 400-1000
   c. 100-400 and greater than 1000
   d. less than 800 and greater than 1000

3. Stridor heard during thoracic auscultation may be differentiated from wheezing by observing that the _____.
   a. frequency (pitch) is much lower than expected with a wheeze
   b. frequency (pitch) is much higher than expected with a wheeze
   c. timing for wheezes is inspiration and for stridor is exhalation
   d. stridor is audible at the mouth without a stethoscope

4. Compared with the unaffected left cranial lobe, auscultation of a right cranial lung lobe that appears completely consolidated with a lobar air bronchogram is expected to produce lung sounds that _____.
   a. are inaudible
   b. are reduced
   c. include wheezing
   d. are increased

5. A mixture of helium and oxygen is less dense than atmospheric gas and when breathed promotes laminar flow within airways. The expected effect on tracheal sounds is _____.
   a. reduction of sound
   b. audible rhonchi
   c. increase in sound
   d. increase in frequency (higher pitch)

Part B

Directions: Part B consists of four unknowns presented on the accompanying website. After determining the correct answers, fill in the appropriate blanks.

1. Sound heard in a dyspneic cat with a history of coughing. _____

2. Lung sounds in a 10-year-old West Highland Terrier with coughing. _____

3. Lung sounds in a 3-year-old asymptomatic Beagle. _____

4. Inspiratory sound in a 12-year-old Labrador Retriever with exercise-induced dyspnea. _____

Canine and Feline Breed Predilections for Heart Disease*

Dog

Breed	Disease	Breed	Disease
Affenpinscher	PDA	Boykin Spaniel	PS Degenerative valve disease
Afghan Hound	DCM	British Bulldog	Arteriovenous fistula Mitral valve disease PS
Airedale	PS Aortic coarctation		
Akita	VSD	Brittany Spaniel	Persistent right aortic arch
Basset Hound	PS VSD	Bullmastiff	PS DCM
Beagle	PS VSD Right bundle branch block Tetralogy of Fallot	Bull Terrier	Mitral valve dysplasia Mitral valve stenosis SAS
Bearded Collie	SAS	Cavalier King Charles Spaniel	Inherited ventricular arrhythmias Right atrial hemangiosarcoma (±pericardial effusion) PDA Degenerative (myxomatous mitral) valve disease Femoral artery occlusion
Bichon Frise	PDA Degenerative valve disease		
Bloodhound	SAS		
Border Terrier	Aortic body tumours VSD		
Boston Terrier	Degenerative valve disease DCM Chemodectoma (±pericardial effusion) PDA	Chihuahua	PDA PS Degenerative valve disease
		Chow Chow	PS VSD
Bouvier des Flandres	SAS	Cocker Spaniel (American, English)	PDA (American, English) PS Degenerative valve disease DCM (American, English) Sick sinus syndrome (American, English)
Boxer	SAS PS ASD DCM Arrhythmogenic right ventricular cardiomyopathy (Boxer cardiomyopathy) Chemodectoma (±pericardial effusion) Endocardial fibroelastosis HCM	Cocker Spaniel, American	Cardiomyopathy PDA
		Collie (Rough and Smooth)	PDA

---

*From Tilley LP, Smith FWK, Jr, Oyama MA, et al, editors: *Manual of canine and feline cardiology*, ed 5, St Louis, 2016, Saunders.

Breed	Disease	Breed	Disease
Dachshund	Degenerative valve disease Mitral valve prolapse Sick sinus syndrome PDA	Golden Retriever	SAS Mitral valve dysplasia Tricuspid valve dysplasia Taurine deficient familial DCM Canine X-linked muscular dystrophy Pericardial effusion, idiopathic Right atrial hemangiosarcoma (±pericardial effusion)
Dalmatian	DCM Mitral valve dysplasia		
Doberman Pinscher	ASD DCM Bundle of His degeneration Persistent right aortic arch		
Dogue de Bordeaux	SAS	Great Dane	Mitral valve dysplasia Tricuspid valve dysplasia SAS PS Persistent right aortic arch DCM Lone atrial fibrillation
English Bulldog (Bulldog)	PS Tetralogy of Fallot VSD SAS Chemodectoma (±pericardial effusion) Mitral valve dysplasia Persistent right aortic arch		
		Great Pyrenees	Tricuspid valve dysplasia
		Greyhound	Persistent right aortic arch
		Husky	VSD
English Sheepdog	DCM	Irish Setter	Persistent right aortic arch DCM Right atrial hemangiosarcoma (±pericardial effusion) Tricuspid dysplasia
English Springer Spaniel	PDA VSD Persistent atrial standstill		
Estrela Mountain Dog	DCM		
		Irish Wolfhound	DCM Lone atrial fibrillation
Fox Terrier	Degenerative valve disease PS (wirehaired and smooth) Tetralogy of Fallot (wirehaired) Persistent right aortic arch (wirehaired and smooth)	Italian Greyhound	Persistent right aortic arch
		Keeshond (Keeshonden)	Conotruncal defects (CTD) includes conal septum, conal VSD, Tetralogy of Fallot, and persistent truncus arteriosus PDA PS Mitral valve dysplasia
French Bulldog	PS		
German Pinscher	Persistent right aortic arch		
German Shepherd	SAS Mitral valve dysplasia Tricuspid valve dysplasia Persistent right aortic arch Inherited ventricular arrhythmia (tachycardia) Right atrial hemangiosarcoma (±pericardial effusion) Infective endocarditis DCM PDA Cardiomyopathy	Kerry Blue Terrier	PDA
		Labrador Retriever	Tricuspid valve dysplasia PDA PS DCM Pericardial effusion, idiopathic Right atrial hemangiosarcoma (±pericardial effusion) Supraventricular tachycardia
German Shorthair Pointer	SAS		

Continued

Breed	Disease	Breed	Disease
Lakeland Terrier	VSD	Rottweiler	SAS
Lhasa Apso	Degenerative valve disease		DCM
			HCM
			Mitral dysplasia
Maltese	PDA	Saint Bernard	DCM
	Mitral dysplasia	Saluki	PDA
Mastiff	Mitral valve dysplasia	Samoyed	PS
	PS		SAS
	Tricuspid valve dysplasia		ASD
Miniature Pinscher	Degenerative valve disease	Schnauzer, Miniature	PS
			PDA
Newfoundland	SAS		Degenerative valve disease
	Mitral valve dysplasia		Sick sinus syndrome
	Mitral valve stenosis	Schnauzer, Standard	PS
	PDA		
	PS	Scottish Deerhound	DCM
	DCM		
	ASD	Scottish Terrier	PS
	VSD	Shetland Sheepdog	PDA
New Zealand Huntaway Dog	DCM		Degenerative valve disease
			Conotruncal heart malformation
Norfolk Terrier	Mitral valve disease		
	Syncope	Shih Tzu	VSD
Old English Sheepdog	Tricuspid valve dysplasia		Degenerative valve disease
	Persistent atrial standstill	Springer Spaniel	DCM
	DCM	Sussex Spaniel	Cardiomyopathy
Pekingese	Degenerative valve disease	Terriers (e.g., Fox Terrier, Mixed Terriers)	PS
			Degenerative valve disease
Pembroke Welsh Corgi	PDA	Weimaraner	Tricuspid valve dysplasia
			Peritoneopericardial diaphragmatic hernia
Pomeranian	PDA		
	Degenerative valve disease	Welsh Corgi (Pembroke)	PDA
	Sick sinus syndrome		
Poodle	PDA (toy and miniature)	West Highland White Terrier	PS
	Degenerative mitral valve disease (toy and miniature)		VSD
			Tetralogy of Fallot
	VSD (toy and miniature)		Degenerative valve disease
	ASD (standard)		Sick sinus syndrome
Portuguese Water Dog	Juvenile DCM	Whippet	Degenerative valve disease
Pug	Atrioventricular block (stenosis of the bundle of His)	Yorkshire Terrier	PDA
			Degenerative valve disease

ASD, Atrial septal defect; DCM, dilated cardiomyopathy; HCM, hypertrophic cardiomyopathy; PDA, patent ductus arteriosus; PS, pulmonic stenosis; SAS, subaortic stenosis; VSD, ventricular septal defect.

Resources

Alroy J, Rush JE, Freeman L, et al: Inherited infantile dilated cardiomyopathy in dogs: genetic, clinical, biochemical, and morphologic findings, *Am J Med Genet* 95(1):57–66, 2000.

Basso C, Fox PR, Meurs KM, et al: Arrhythmogenic right ventricular cardiomyopathy causing sudden cardiac death in boxer dogs: a new animal model of human disease, *Circulation* 109(9):1180–1185, 2004. e-pub: March 1, 2004.

Bélanger MC, Ouellet M, Queney G, et al: Taurine-deficient dilated cardiomyopathy in a family of Golden Retrievers, *JAAHA* 41:284–291, 2005.

Chetboul V, Charles V, et al: Retrospective study of 156 atrial septal defects in dogs and cats, *J Vet Med A Physiol Pathol Clin Med* 53(4):179–184, 2006.

Chetboul V, Trolle JM, et al: Congenital heart diseases in the boxer dog: a retrospective study of 105 cases (1998-2005), *J Vet Med A Physiol Pathol Clin Med* 53(7):346–351, 2006.

Dambach DM, Lannon A, Sleeper MM, et al: Familial dilated cardiomyopathy of young Portuguese water dogs, *J Vet Intern Med* 13(1):65–71, 1999.

Fox PR, Sisson D, Moïse NS, editors: *Textbook of canine and feline cardiology,* ed 2, Philadelphia 1999, WB Saunders.

Gordon SG, Saunders AB, et al: Atrial septal defects in an extended family of standard poodles. In *Proceedings,* 2006, The Annual ACVIM Forum, p 730.

Gunby JM, Hardie RJ, Bjorling DE: Investigation of the potential heritability of persistent right aortic arch in Greyhounds, *J Am Vet Med Assoc* 224(7):1120–1122, 2004.

Hyun C, Lavulo L: Congenital heart diseases in small animals. I. Genetic pathways and potential candidate genes, *Vet J* 171(2):245–255, 2006. Comment in *Vet J* 171(2):195–197, 2006.

Hyun C, Park IC: Congenital heart diseases in small animals. II. Potential genetic aetiologies based on human genetic studies, *Vet J* 171(2):256–262, 2006. Comment in *Vet J* 171(2):195–197, 2006.

Kittleson MD, Kienle RD, editors: *Small animal cardiovascular medicine,* Philadelphia, 1998, Mosby.

MacDonald KA: Congenital heart diseases of puppies and kittens, *Vet Clin North Am Small Anim Pract* 36(3):503–531, 2006.

Meurs KM: Inherited heart disease in the dog. In *Proceedings,* 2003, Tufts Genetics Symposium, 2003.

Meurs KM: Update on Boxer arrhythmogenic right ventricular cardiomyopathy (ARVC). In *Proceedings,* 2005, The Annual ACVIM Forum, p 106.

Meurs KM, Fox PR, Nogard M, et al: A prospective genetic evaluation of familial dilated cardiomyopathy in the Doberman Pinscher, *J Vet Intern Med* 21:1016–1020, 2007.

Meurs KM, Spier AW, Miller MW, et al: Familial ventricular arrhythmias in boxers, *J Vet Intern Med* 13(5):437–439, 1999.

Meurs KM, Spier AW, Wright NA, et al: Comparison of the effects of four antiarrhythmic treatments for familial ventricular arrhythmias in Boxers, *J Am Vet Med Assoc* 221(4):522–527, 2002.

Moïse NS: Update on inherited arrhythmias in German Shepherds. In *Proceedings,* 2005, The Annual ACVIM Forum, pp 67–68.

Olsen LH, Fredholm M, Pedersen HD: Epidemiology and inheritance of mitral valve prolapse in Dachshunds, *J Vet Intern Med* 13(5):448–456, 1999.

Parker HG, Meurs KM, Ostrander EA: Finding cardiovascular disease genes in the dog, *J Vet Cardiol* 8:115–127, 2006.

Phillip, U et al. A rare form of persistent right aorta arch in linkage disequilibrium with the DiGeorge critical region on CFA26 in German Pinschers, *J Hered* 102(51):S68–S73, 2011.

Schober KE, Baade H: Doppler echocardiographic prediction of pulmonary hypertension in West Highland white terriers with chronic pulmonary disease, *J Vet Intern Med* 20:912–920, 2006.

Spier AW, Meurs KM, Muir WW, et al: Correlation of QT dispersion with indices used to evaluate the severity of familial ventricular arrhythmias in Boxers, *Am J Vet Res* 62(9):1481–1485, 2001.

Tidholm A: Retrospective study of congenital heart defects in 151 dogs, *J Small Anim Pract* 38(3):94–98, 2006.

Vollmar AC, Fox PR: Assessment of cardiovascular diseases in 527 Boxers. In *Proceedings,* 2005, The Annual ACVIM Forum, p 65.

Vollmar AC, Trötschel C: Cardiomyopathy in Irish Wolfhounds. In *Proceedings,* 2005, The Annual ACVIM Forum, p 66.

Werner P, Raducha MG, Prociuk U, et al: The Keeshond defect in cardiac conotruncal development is oligogenic, *Human Genet* 116(5):368–377, 2005. e-pub: Feb 12, 2005.

Cat

Breed	Condition	Breed	Condition
Abysssinian	Subvalvular pulmonary stenosis	Persian	Systemic hypertension Septal defect
Birman	Systemic hypertension	Ragdoll	HCM
British Shorthair	HCM Septal defect	Siamese	Systemic hypertension Septal defect
Burmese	Septal defect Congenital heart defect		Congenital heart defect Mitral valve stenosis PDA
Chartreux	Septal defect Systemic hypertension		SAS Supravalvular aortic stenosis
Devon Rex	Subvalvular pulmonary stenosis		Tetralogy of Fallot Tricuspid stenosis
Maine Coon	HCM Septal defect	Siberian	HCM
		Sphynx	HCM
Norwegian Forest Cat	HCM		MVD

HCM, Hypertrophic cardiomyopathy; *MVD,* mitral valve dysplasia; *PDA,* patent ductus arteriosus; *SAS,* subaortic stenosis..

Genetic and Health Databases and Resources Accessed

Bell JS, Cavanagh KE, Tilley LP, Smith FWK: *Veterinary medical guide to dog and cat breeds,* Jackson, WY, 2012, Teton NewMedia.

Cambridge Veterinary School Database: http://www.vet.cam.ac.uk/idid.

Chetboul V, et al: Prospective echocardiographic and tissue Doppler screening of a large Sphynx cat population: reference ranges, heart disease prevalence and genetic aspects, *J Vet Cardiol* 14(4):497–509, 2012.

National Institutes of Health Library: http://www.ncbi.nlm.nih.gov/pmc.

Online Mendelian Inheritance in Animals: http://omia.angis.org.au/home.

Online Mendelian Inheritance in Man: http://www.ncbi.nlm.nih.gov/omim.

PubMed Literature Database: http://www.ncbi.nlm.nih.gov/pubmed.

Sargan DR: IDID: inherited diseases in dogs: web-based information for canine inherited disease genetics, *Mamm Genome* 15(6):503–506, 2004.

University of Australia Faculty of Veterinary Medicine Database (LIDA): http://sydney.edu.au/vetscience/lida.

UPEI Canine Inherited Disorders Database: http://www.upei.ca/~cidd/intro.htm.

Recommended Readings

Cote E, MacDonald KA, Meurs KM, et al, editors: Heart murmurs and gallop heart sounds. In *Feline cardiology*, West Sussex, UK, 2011, Wiley-Blackwell.

Cote E, Manning AM, Emerson D, et al: Assessment of the prevalence of heart murmurs in overtly healthy cats, *J Am Vet Med Assoc* 225:384, 2004.

Dennis S: Sound advice for heart murmurs, *J Small Anim Pract* 54:443, 2013.

Erickson B: *Heart sounds and murmurs: across the lifespan*, ed 4, St Louis, 2003, Mosby.

Fang JC, O'Gara PT: The history and physical examination: an evidence-based approach. In Bonow RO, Mann DL, Zipes DP, et al, editors: *Braunwald's heart disease: a textbook of cardiovascular medicine*, ed 9, Philadelphia, 2012, Saunders.

Gompf RE: The history and physical examination. In Tilley LP, Smith FWK, Oyama MA, et al, editors: *Manual of canine and feline cardiology*, ed 4, St Louis, 2001, Saunders.

Kittleson MD, Kienle RD: Signalment, history, and physical examination. In Kittleson MD, Kienle RD, editors: *Small animal cardiovascular medicine*, St Louis, 1998, Mosby.

Kotlikoff MI, Gillespie JR: Lung sounds in veterinary medicine. I. Terminology and mechanisms of sound production, *Comp Cont Educ Pract Vet* 5(8;9):634–639, 1983.

Kotlikoff MI, Gillespie JR: Lung sounds in veterinary medicine. II. Deriving clinical information from lung sounds, *Comp Cont Educ Pract Vet* 6(5):462–467, 1984.

Kvart C, Häggström J: *Cardiac auscultation and phonocardiography in dogs, horses, and cats*, Uppsala, Sweden, 2002, TK i Uppsala AB.

Naylor JM: *Art of bovine auscultation*, Oxford, 2004, Blackwell.

Naylor JM: *The art of equine auscultation: an interactive guide* (CD-ROM for Windows), Oxford, 2004, Blackwell.

Prosek R: Abnormal heart sounds and heart murmurs. In Ettinger SJ, Feldman EC, editors: *A textbook of veterinary internal medicine*, ed 7, Philadelphia, 2010, Saunders.

Rishniw M, Thomas WP: Dynamic right ventricular outflow obstruction: a new cause of systolic murmurs in cats, *J Vet Intern Med* 16(5):547, 2002.

Roudebush P: Lung sounds, *J Am Vet Med Assoc* 181:122, 1982.

Sisson D, Ettinger SJ: The physical examination. In Fox PR, Sisson D, Moise NS, editors: *Textbook of canine and feline cardiology*, ed 2, Philadelphia, 1999, Saunders.

Stein E, Delman A: *Rapid interpretation of heart sounds and murmurs*, ed 3, Philadelphia, 1990, Lea & Febiger.

Tilkian AG, Conover MB: *Understanding heart sounds and murmurs: with an introduction to lung sounds*, ed 4, Philadelphia, 2001, Saunders.

Tilley LP, Smith FWK, editors: *Blackwell's five-minute veterinary consult: canine and feline*, ed 5, West Sussex, UK, 2011, Wiley-Blackwell.

Wilkins RL: *Fundamentals of lung and heart sounds*, ed 3, St Louis, 2004, Mosby.

APPENDIX 3

Answers to Pretests and Posttests

Pretests

Answers to Pretest 1
1. c
2. d
3. a
4. c
5. b
6. b
7. d
8. d
9. a
10. d

Answers to Pretest 2
1. d
2. a
3. c
4. d
5. b
6. c

7. d
8. d
9. d
10. d

Answers to Pretest 3
1. b
2. c
3. d
4. b
5. a

Answers to Pretest 4
1. c
2. a
3. b
4. c
5. d

Posttests

Answers to Posttest 1
Part A
1. True
2. False
3. False
4. True
5. True
6. True
7. True
8. False
9. False
10. True

Part B
1. Quadruple rhythm
2. Aortic ejection sound
3. Summation sound

4. "Fixed" splitting of S_2
5. Third heart sound (S_3)
6. Midsystolic clicks
7. Pulmonic ejection sound
8. Fourth heart sound (S_4)
9. Physiologic splitting of S_2
10. Persistent splitting of S_2

Answers to Posttest 2
Part A
1. a
2. d
3. b
4. c
5. b
6. d

7. a
8. d
9. d
10. d

Part B

1. Systolic ejection murmur of aortic stenosis
2. Continuous or "machinery" murmur of patent ductus arteriosus
3. To-and-fro murmur of aortic stenosis and regurgitation
4. Holosystolic murmur of myxomatous degeneration of the mitral valve
5. Holosystolic murmur with a heart rate of 210 beats/min. The cat is probably in heart failure and needs an echocardiogram as well as a chest radiograph to further define the defect present.

Answers to Posttest 3

Part A

1. b
2. a
3. a
4. d
5. c

Part B

1. Atrial fibrillation
2. Sinus arrhythmia
3. Ventricular tachycardia based on ECG. Atrial tachycardia would also be a differential diagnosis based on auscultation alone. The history in this case supports traumatic myocarditis, so ventricular tachycardia would be more likely. If split heart sounds were recognized, this supports an auscultatory diagnosis of ventricular tachycardia; however, splitting is only occasionally recognized in clinical cases. An ECG is needed for a definitive diagnosis.
4. Sinus arrhythmia with premature ventricular contractions. The compensatory pause following the premature beats suggests a ventricular origin, as does splitting of the heart sounds, but again an ECG is needed to confirm the origin of the premature beats heard.

Answers to Posttest 4

Part A

1. c
2. b
3. d
4. d
5. a

Part B

1. Wheeze
2. Crackles
3. Normal breath sounds
4. Inspiratory stridor caused by laryngeal paralysis

Page numbers followed by *f, t,* and *b* indicate figures, tables, and boxes, respectively.

Printed and bound by CPI Group (UK) Ltd, Croydon, CR0 4YY

03/10/2024

01040364-0003